The Practice of Tui Na

of related interest

Tui Na
A Manual of Chinese Massage Therapy
Sarah Pritchard
ISBN 978 1 84819 269 0
eISBN 978 0 85701 218 0

Tuina/Massage Manipulations
Basic Principles and Techniques
Chief Editor: Li Jiangshan
ISBN 978 1 78592 997 7
eISBN 978 0 85701 046 9

Daoist Reflections from Scholar Sage
Damo Mitchell and his students
ISBN 978 1 84819 321 5
eISBN 978 0 85701 274 6

Heavenly Streams
Meridian Theory in Nei Gong
Damo Mitchell
Foreword by Robert Aspell
ISBN 978 1 84819 116 7
eISBN 978 0 85701 092 6

The Practice of

TUI NA

Principles, Diagnostics and Working
with the Sinew Channels

ROB ASPELL

Foreword by Damo Mitchell
Illustrations by Spencer Hill and Rob Aspell

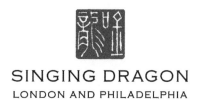

SINGING DRAGON
LONDON AND PHILADELPHIA

First published in 2019
by Singing Dragon
an imprint of Jessica Kingsley Publishers
73 Collier Street
London N1 9BE, UK
and
400 Market Street, Suite 400
Philadelphia, PA 19106, USA

www.singingdragon.com

Library of Congress Cataloging in Publication Data
A CIP catalog record for this book is available from the Library of Congress

British Library Cataloguing in Publication Data
A CIP catalogue record for this book is available from the British Library

ISBN 978 1 84819 412 0
eISBN 978 0 85701 370 5

Printed and bound in Great Britain

Contents

Section 2: Diagnostics of Tui Na

Section 3: Hand Techniques

Section 4: Treatment Guidelines

Foreword

Mastery of Tui Na is a difficult attainment for sure; although it may be fairly simple to begin learning some individual techniques, it can take a person a lifetime to truly embody the highest levels of Tui Na practice. When studying in Asia, it can be impressive enough to see the professional Tui Na practitioners at work but then, if you have the good fortune to meet a real master of the art, it can be mind-blowing to see just how far the practice can be taken. It is often the case that, in Chinese Medicine, the people who reach the pinnacle of the practice have been born into a family of practitioners and represent the latest generation of their family in the medical arts. The therapeutic touch of Tui Na begins mechanical, as with any other form of bodywork, but with time progresses to something quite beyond what may be rationally explained. To the traditional Chinese, they will simply say that it is down to the nature of the practitioners' Qi and the quality of their Gong Fu (skill developed over time).

In modern times, the kind of dedication required for this kind of skill level can seem daunting as we are often looking for quick routes into becoming an 'expert', but this is often because we don't view arts such as Tui Na in the correct light. To the ancient Chinese, each of their arts was considered not just a practice in its own right or a medical modality, but rather as a form of personal cultivation. At the highest levels of development, an art such as Tui Na could even become a spiritual practice that could, according to ancient belief systems, lead a person to an inner awakening. This is because any personal endeavour, if taken to its highest level, would begin to evolve into a form of meditation that could transform the mindset of the practitioner as well as the inner state of the patient, in the case of a practice such as Tui Na.

As with all practices, we should begin with theory and then some methods. These are what the Chinese call 'Fa', techniques that we have to develop so that we have the required tools for what we do. After this we have the lengthy stage of developing our 'Fa' into what are known as 'Gong'. Gong is often translated as meaning 'skill' but this translation hardly does the term justice. It is higher than a skill; it is the process of taking any technique, method or practice and developing it over a long period of time until it becomes an inherent part of our very being, a 'quality' that is built into what we do and who we are. Understanding this process can give us a window into what it actually means for a practice to become a form of personal cultivation. As with almost all Chinese Arts, the enigmatic concept/actuality of Qi plays a large part in this process, and so it has always been the traditional way that Tui Na practitioners, and indeed proponents of all

Chinese medical modalities, developed and maintained a regular practice of Qi Gong alongside their clinical work. All of these elements together would help to develop the practitioner and ultimately also provide a higher quality treatment to the sick.

Sadly, in modern times, it is often the case that much of what is written above is either unknown or not taken into consideration when people begin to learn an art such as Tui Na. It is my opinion that it is largely down to a simple lack of information being available in the West to students and practitioners of Tui Na alike. This is where this book by my dear friend Rob Aspell comes in. Rob has presented here, in *The Practice of Tui Na: Principles, Diagnostics and Working with the Sinew Channels*, a strong philosophical and practical groundwork for the new student entering into a practice of Tui Na as well as an insightful and detailed text that will benefit longer-term practitioners of Chinese medical bodywork. I was delighted to find in the book clear guidance on the 'virtues' of Tui Na, the nature of skill development and an importance placed on mental qualities and internal development as well as clear instruction on technique and application of Tui Na to specific physical and psychological conditions. This is a book for the 'cultivator' of Tui Na, and will serve to set somebody on the path to mastery if they apply these teachings in their clinical practice.

A further aspect of Tui Na practice that is often overlooked is the fact that it is based on similar but not identical theories to Acupuncture. Whilst both systems use channels and Acupuncture points to achieve therapeutic effect, Tui Na actually uses a different set of channels to Acupuncture. Rather than simply applying some hand techniques with Acupuncture theory, Tui Na should be learned in conjunction with the all-important Sinew channels. Although most Chinese medical practitioners will be familiar with the Sinew channels, it is often the case that they are given an almost cursory level of study compared to the Organ channel system in most modern Chinese Medicine schools. Rob has clearly and succinctly discussed the nature of the Sinew channels, their diagnosis and usage in treatment through Tui Na methodologies in this book; this, alone, should be enough to make the book stand out from others in the field, and hopefully many practitioners of Chinese Medicine will benefit from the information Rob is imparting here.

I have known Rob for quite a number of years now. We met through Chinese Medicine, have travelled together in China, have shared ideas and concepts around these arts, and now I have the honour of teaching alongside him in our own college of Chinese Medicine. His skill level is very high and his knowledge broad. This is, in part, due to his training, but also because he is somebody who lives and breathes Chinese Medicine as a form of cultivation, as discussed above. Not content with simply learning a method, he always has to take it further and see how it can be developed and applied in more effective ways. Despite this need to always develop his practice, he stays close to the root of his art, with consistent study of the classical texts of Chinese Medicine and traditional methods of past masters. I am, by the nature of who I am, very picky with regards to who I endorse and, most certainly, who I choose to teach alongside. These arts are a precious treasure that deserve to be treated with respect and passed on with due care. This means that only those with a high level of skill and passion for a practice such as Tui Na should be the ones passing on teachings such as those contained within this book, and I can safely say that I know Rob Aspell to be just such a person. I hope this book is wide-reaching and influences Chinese medical practice in the beneficial manner that I know it should.

Damo Mitchell, author of *A Comprehensive Guide to Daoist Nei Gong*
Portugal, September 2018

Acknowledgements

This book could not exist without the generosity of the teachers and practitioners who have shared with me their knowledge of Tui Na, and, of course, Chinese Medicine and the Chinese Arts. It would also not have been possible without the enthusiasm of the efforts of my students, past and present – so thank you to all of my teachers and students for being both my motivation and my inspiration, and for making it so enjoyable to practise and share my passion for Chinese Medicine. For this I am truly grateful.

I would next like to give huge thanks and acknowledgement to fellow Chinese Medicine practitioner and good friend Matthew Budd, for his contributions to the diagnostics section of this book, and for his invaluable and thought-provoking ideas about Chinese Medicine and bodywork (usually whilst eating Thai food somewhere in Chester) – great work exploring and pushing the boundaries of modern bodywork whilst remaining rooted within the solid foundations of Chinese Medicine.

Thank you very much to all those who have helped me with the writing of this book, including Spencer Hill for his excellent illustrations and artistic direction, Vicky Oakey for transcribing one of our classes that contributed to some of the information in this book, and both Ela Pekalska and Vicky Oakey (again) for taking the time to read through my writings (as Tui Na practitioners themselves) and helping me to edit the final book – this book would not have been as complete without you all!

A massive thank you also to my friend Paul Beasant for the many fun times over the years we spent studying, practising and teaching Tui Na together, where we learned to expect the unexpected – there was *never* a dull moment!

I also give my deepest gratitude to my good friend and teaching partner Damo Mitchell, for not only writing the Foreword to this book, but also for the inspiration in striving to truly connect with the understandings of classical Chinese and Daoist Medicine, and for the incredible times we have had teaching Chinese Medicine and visiting Asia together.

Last but not least, thank you also to all at Singing Dragon for giving me the opportunity to write this book, and in particular Claire Wilson for helping me to realise my ideas and supporting me throughout.

Introduction

First, Tui Na is a *lot* more than just 'massage' – it is a whole stand-alone medical system, and is one of the oldest methods of treatment still used today, becoming the foundation of many more modern therapies. Tui Na is one of the 'Four Pillars' of Chinese Medicine (alongside Acupuncture, Herbal Medicine and Qi Gong), and despite often being translated as 'Chinese Medical Massage', it is a form of bodywork that includes acupressure, massage techniques, assisted stretching and joint mobilisations or adjustments that are all based on the key medical principles and diagnostics of the Classics of Chinese Medicine.

As with any type of therapy, it is important to understand that it is the principles and diagnostics that make the therapy, and not simply the techniques. It is about understanding what needs to be done and why, in addition to understanding ways in which to do it. For instance, Tui Na contains joint manipulations that are similar to Chiropractic practice or Osteopathy; however, we are not chiropractors or osteopaths. It contains techniques such as 'kneading' and 'pressing' that are similar to Western massage, yet we are not massage therapists. Tui Na also contains stretches that have the appearance of Yoga postures, yet we are not Yoga teachers. This is because it is the principles behind a system that define the system.

Defining systems

It is not the *techniques*, but the *principles* behind a system that define the system.

Tui Na is becoming increasingly popular within the West, and even within China there seems to be a new respect for Tui Na within the more modern Chinese Medicine hospitals and recent Chinese Medicine conferences. With this come more and more courses offering Tui Na as either stand-alone courses or as part of other courses, and awareness of Tui Na is becoming greater. Although Tui Na hand techniques and treatment 'protocols' are generally taught well, the understanding of Tui Na as a stand-alone medical system is not. This is sad, because a system that loses its principles becomes empty and diluted, and soon it will indeed become just another 'massage' therapy.

Easily one of the biggest mistakes within the teachings of Tui Na is that it is treated as merely an adjunct to more popular Chinese Medicine modalities such as Acupuncture and/or Herbal Medicine, or even that Tui Na is simply a 'hands-on' version of Acupuncture. Whereas this is absolutely fine if it is indeed going to be used as an 'adjunct' to these therapies, Tui Na has its own principles in its own right that should be understood if it is to be used alone. While based on the core principles of the Chinese Medicine model (as almost all Chinese Arts are, including Qi Gong, Martial Arts, and even Feng Shui), there are major differences and perspectives that need to be understood in order to truly understand how to treat using Tui Na beyond simply musculoskeletal conditions. For example, one of the most common misinterpretations of Tui Na is that it uses the same channel system as Acupuncture – the Primary channels. However, perhaps the most important aspect of Tui Na is to understand the *Sinew* channels.

Even when some students or practitioners realise the importance of the Sinew channels, it is often misunderstood that they follow the same principles as the Primary channels and that only the pathways are slightly different. In fact, the principles behind the Sinew channels, including their individual functions, the order and direction in which they flow and their behaviours are almost entirely different to those of the channels that are utilised within Acupuncture. I could go as bold as to say that, not understanding the Sinew channels in the way that they are intended is like a surgeon not understanding anatomy! For this reason, understanding the Sinew channels forms a major part of this book, and is vital in knowing how to use Tui Na to its full potential beyond a musculoskeletal therapy.

Core principles

Only by having a deep understanding of the core principles and practice of Tui Na can we become *broadminded* and *lateral thinking* in our diagnosis, and completely *spontaneous* in our treatment. This helps to minimise our limits.

Another important factor in learning a 'hands-on' or 'practical' modality is the importance of understanding the theory that goes with it – it will simply make your practice better! Within Chinese Medicine, we learn about what is known as the Yi (意), which can be interpreted as both the mind, awareness and our intellect (as well as other aspects of the psyche, discussed later in this book). Knowing the importance of engaging and training the Yi in regards to technique quality and effectiveness also demonstrates the importance of understanding the theories and principles that underpin any physical practice. Within the Chinese Arts, it is thought to be important to 'feed' and 'train' the Yi with knowledge of the subject, and therefore to allow the Yi to develop and grow in a certain way in order to gain greater focus and intent whilst performing the physical aspect of the specific art. This is why it is important to have a thorough understanding of the theoretical aspect of *any* practice in addition to the practical aspect.

This book was written with the above in mind to act as both a companion to entirely new students whilst studying on a hands-on practical course in Tui Na, in addition to hopefully providing greater understanding and to spark further interest to already qualified Chinese Medicine and Tui Na practitioners.

The book has been split into four main sections:

- Section 1: Foundations of Tui Na

- Section 2: Diagnostics of Tui Na

- Section 3: Hand Techniques

- Section 4: Treatment Guidelines

Just like reference books on other Chinese Medicine subjects, this book does not need to be read front to back or page by page. It has been written in a way that it can be picked up quickly and used practically. I hope that you enjoy learning from this book, and that it both helps your Tui Na practice and sparks greater interest in Chinese Medicine as a whole. Thank you for reading!

FOUNDATIONS OF TUI NA

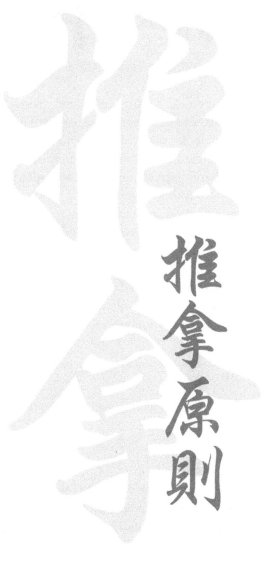

Chapter 1

Introduction to Tui Na

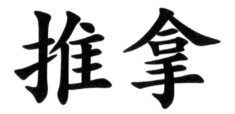

Chinese characters for Tui (推) Na (拿)

The terms 'Tui' and 'Na' literally mean 'to push' and 'to grasp' respectively, and are, in fact, also the names of two of the core techniques that are used within the practice of Tui Na. The reason that it was chosen to be called Tui Na, and not named after any of the other techniques such as An Rou or even An Tui was not simply by coincidence, but because each and every technique that is used within Tui Na should include the energetics of either Tui (to push in) or Na (to take hold, grasp or to draw out). They essentially reflect the importance of the concept of Yin and Yang within Tui Na, with Tui being the Yang to the Yin of Na (again, Yang is to push in whereas Yin would be to grasp and to draw out). It is important to understand this concept from the beginning, as when performing each technique, the student or practitioner's intent and awareness are just as important as the physical techniques themselves. Understanding that with every technique you are either applying the Yang intent of 'pushing into the body', the Yin intent of 'pulling out of the body', or a combination of the two, is essential.

Pushing and grasping

Every technique within Tui Na should contain elements of either *Tui* or *Na*, or a combination of both.

Other traditional bodywork therapies do exist in China, such as An Mo (按摩, pressing and rubbing), An Qiao (按蹻, pressing and stepping) and Zhi Ya (指壓, acupressure). However, Tui Na is the only bodywork therapy that is considered as being medical, and the only major bodywork therapy that follows the vast principles and diagnostics of Chinese Medicine.

The origins of Tui Na date back to long before any other form of Chinese Medicine, and bodywork in general is thought to possibly outdate any other form of medicine still practised today. Early bodywork was thought to have derived from instinctual methods – we all feel the urge to gently rub our abdomen if there is discomfort or bloating, or quickly rub an injured limb to help ease the pain. It was then thought to have developed beyond 'instinctual methods' within the schools of Martial Arts, and also within larger labouring communities. This was understandably due to the increased likelihood of soft tissue injuries and joint dislocations caused by the harsher way of living. During this time, a major focus was also placed on paediatric disorders and internal disorders for the elderly (most commonly, digestive disorders).

The earliest archaeological findings of Tui Na date back to before the Shang Dynasty, which began at around 1800 BC. Tui Na is also listed as one of the key medical treatment methods within the *Huang Di Nei Jing* (*Yellow Emperor's Classic of Internal Medicine*), which is one of the earliest Chinese medical texts, and one of the earliest medical texts in the world. Here, a number of Tui Na techniques and their actions are described alongside the use of Tui Na as a palpation diagnostic method. There is even evidence of a book called *Huang Di Qi Bo An Mo Shi Juan* (*Ten Volumes of Massage by Huang Di and Qi Bo*) that was written at the same time as the *Nei Jing*, although unfortunately only records of its existence remain and the actual book has been lost.

Although the origins of Tui Na date back thousands of years, it wasn't until around the Ming Dynasty (around 1400 AD) that it was given the name 'Tui Na'. This was so that it could be distinguished from other forms of bodywork due to its much higher technical level and in-depth medical principles, which, during this time, were rapidly advancing. In modern times, Tui Na is practised within Chinese Medicine hospitals as a major part of the healthcare system, much in the same way that Physiotherapy and Osteopathy is used in the West.

Core principles of Tui Na

The core principles of Tui Na are based on the key fundamental theories and diagnostics of Chinese Medicine. Ultimately, Tui Na should not simply be viewed as a massage or a bodywork therapy, but rather as a whole medical system that can be used to treat the whole body for both external and internal conditions. What is important to understand is that it is not knowing how to perform the techniques that make you a Tui Na practitioner, but knowing the principles behind what we do as Tui Na practitioners. It is essential that the practitioner keeps in mind these principles, rather than mindlessly performing the hand techniques that make up only part of the system.

For example, Tui Na contains many joint manipulations that are similar to Osteopathy, although this does not make us osteopaths because we do not keep to the fundamental principles of Osteopathy. Tui Na contains many massage techniques that are similar to Western Sports Massage, although we are not Sports Massage therapists because we do not follow their principles. It is the principles of Chinese Medicine that set Tui Na apart from other bodywork therapies, not the techniques. Over the following pages I will discuss the main principles of Chinese Medicine from a Tui Na perspective that should be adhered to in order to treat effectively both external (channels and collaterals) and internal (organ system-related) medical conditions.

Note: The following pages will assume that the reader has a basic grasp of the fundamental theories and concepts of Chinese Medicine, and will not go into detail regarding these theories. A good introduction to Chinese Medicine can be found, for instance, in *Basic Theories of Traditional Chinese Medicine* by Cheng Xinnong, Zhu Bing and Wang Hongcai.

Balancing Yin and Yang

From Chinese Medicine theory, we know that Yin and Yang are the laws of opposite – mutual support and consumption, interdependence and intertransformation. Every aspect of the natural world can be explained through the concept of Yin and Yang, and this theory helps us to understand the body in a way that is clear and simple. Chinese Medicine is about understanding that the body is in chaos and constant flux, and recognising patterns of the body to enable us to make sense of and to balance this chaos. The Yin and Yang theory is one of many concepts that help us to understand that, and put into a context that can be worked with.

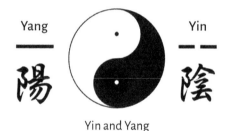

Yin and Yang

Balancing Yin and Yang is one of the most fundamentally important aspects of treatment within Chinese Medicine. In regards to the body and wellbeing, it is necessary for the body to maintain equilibrium in function – a balance between hypoactivity and hyperactivity, weakness and tension, activity and rest. In regards to Tui Na, we can view Yang as tension, heat, hyperactivity or excess patterns, whereas we can view Yin as too relaxed or atrophied, cold, hypoactivity or patterns of deficiency. In terms of techniques, we can view Yang as being quick, powerful and dispersing, with Yin as being slow, gentle and nourishing. We can also view Yang as being superficial with Yin as being deep, yet Yang as being strong and Yin as being soft.

Yang	Yin
Tui	Na
Tension	Flaccidity
Powerful	Gentle
Heat	Cold

Hyperactivity	Hypoactivity
Excessive	Deficient
Quick	Slow
Dispersing	Gathering
Superficial	Deep
Strong	Soft
Qi	Blood

For the body to remain in good health, we are looking for the equal balance between strength (Yang) and relaxation (Yin), and we achieve this by altering the state of each technique and therefore the state of the body's tissues and energy system. Rou Fa (kneading), for example, can be used fast and strong to help break down tissue, or slow and gentle to help build strength and bring nourishment (through Qi and Blood) to an area. Manipulations should also be chosen appropriately according to the patient's constitution. If a patient is very Yin (soft, weak, deficient), we should strengthen the body by using gentle, nourishing techniques to build the Qi and Blood. If a patient is very Yang (too much tension), we should break down the tension using stronger techniques to help disperse stagnation and improve circulation to the tissues.

Regulating the Zang Fu (internal organs)

Tui Na is essentially an external therapy, and although it does *not* directly affect the internal organs, it has the ability to treat internally (meaning it can treat and regulate the functioning of the internal organs of the body). Tui Na works directly with the Sinew channels (discussed later in this section) and the Wei Qi (衛氣), which, in turn, affects the Primary channels and the flow of Ying Qi (營氣) to the internal pathways, and therefore the Zang Fu organs. The channel systems not only include the physical systems of the body (such as the skin, circulatory, nervous, sinews and others), but are also energetic extensions of the organs, directing Qi and Blood to and from the organs and connecting the body as a whole. Think of it as like the transport and road network of a country connecting towns and cities. By regulating the flow of Qi and Blood to the internal organs via the channel system, and ensuring that there are no blockages of the internal pathways, the body can begin to self-regulate and heal itself from within. What's more, by using acupressure to individually activate specific acupoints along the Primary channels, the practitioner can use the functions of both the body's physical and energetic system to regulate the body, as would an acupuncturist or herbalist. Many techniques involve opening the channels by creating space within them and relaxing the tissues around them to reduce and remove stagnation, enabling the Qi and Blood to flow smoothly to nourish the internal organs. In order to treat internally, however, it is important to understand the theories and diagnostics of Chinese Medicine, with a focus on the relationships between the Zang Fu organs themselves, and their relationships with the Vital Substances and their circulation.

Opening and dredging the channels, and promoting the circulation of Qi, Blood and Body Fluids

Opening the channels means to create expansion and space so that the Vital Substances can move through them, whereas dredging (discussed later in this section, see 'The nine therapeutic methods of Tui Na' in Chapter 2) refers to the clearing of a channel, and in some cases, of a joint. Dredging, in the same way as physically dredging a river, is used in order to clear a channel and remove any unwanted blockages, pathogens or debris from a channel and/or joint. Through general daily activities, the body contracts and develops pathogens and debris that build up within the channels and collaterals. The channels and collaterals are designed to deal with and purge these pathogens from the body on a continual basis. However, over time and due to inefficiency of the body (perhaps due to the influences of lifestyle or poor health), pathogens and debris can build up within the channels, making it difficult for the body to remove and expel them by itself. This will cause obstruction within the channels, and affect the circulation of Qi and Blood. Once the channels and collaterals are clear of obstruction, Qi and Blood are able to move freely and nourish the tissues and organs of the body, with the body once again being able to self-regulate, therefore allowing healing in addition to injury prevention.

Calming the Shen (mind) and releasing the emotions

The topic of Shen is a hugely important yet intricate aspect of Chinese Medicine, essentially explaining the complexities of the human psyche, so I will keep it straightforward here and use the term 'Shen' simply to refer to the mind as a whole (more details on the Shen can be found in Section 4). It should be noted that when discussing the Shen, we are also essentially discussing the emotional state of the mind, which is fundamentally an energetic by-product and manifestation of the interactions within the Shen that is potentially harmful. It is increasingly becoming accepted within modern medicine that the Shen (mind) is affected by the body, and vice versa; there are arguably no physical symptoms that do not affect the Shen, and no emotional disorders that do not produce physical manifestations.

For instance, if I were to suffer from chronic pain, this would begin to make me feel certain emotions such as frustration, irritability or even sadness and grief (for various reasons). What's more, the pain will disrupt my sleep, which will go on to create further emotional distress as the Shen is unable to rest. Conversely, if I were to feel emotions such as stress and anxiety over a period of time, it may eventually give rise to tightness in the chest or to a knotted feeling in my abdomen. This clearly shows the relationship between emotions and the physical tissues of our body. The ability for the Shen to transform the tissues of the body by the power of thought alone is amazing; however, this transformation can work both ways, for good and for bad. Within Chinese Medicine, the Shen and the emotions are the main root of disease.

The way that the body works and reacts is this – if one feels emotions such as stress or anxiety, the muscles of the chest, shoulders and neck can begin to tighten. Tension in the connective tissue within the chest, shoulders and neck is a common complaint from patients experiencing stress and anxiety. This is essentially a defence mechanism of the body caused by the reaction of the Wei Qi and the Sinew channels (acting as the body's protection) when there is a perceived feeling of threat; the exterior of the body is protecting the internal organs. The issue lies with most people being unable to return from this reaction, which then has a detrimental effect in the long term. This will then affect the functioning of the organs within the area, mainly the Lungs and the Heart in this instance.

Another issue is that this mechanism works both ways, and if the patient experiences tension in the chest, neck or shoulders (perhaps due to poor posture or lifestyle), over time the body may begin to *think* that there is a threat and give rise to emotions such as anxiety or stress due to the obstruction of Qi and Blood. The same can be said about emotions such as sadness and melancholy – these emotions are said to cause a deficiency of Qi within the chest, therefore causing a collapse in the upright posture of the chest, whereas a collapse in the upright posture around the chest (perhaps due to working conditions such as being sat at a computer) can also create the feeling of sadness and melancholy due to the association between the two and the flow of Qi and Blood within the area.

In regards to calming the Shen and releasing emotions, the most effective way is always going to be using techniques that cultivate the mind directly, such as meditation and mindfulness. However, due to the mind and body being so closely connected and essentially different manifestations of the same thing, calming the Shen can also be done very effectively through the use of bodywork such as Tui Na.

We do this by aligning the body tissues and structure to ensure that everything is physically where and how it should be, therefore allowing the Qi and Blood to flow smoothly and for the Shen to move as it should. By enabling the Qi and Blood to flow smoothly, and by releasing physical tension from the body to allow the Sinew channels to readjust and relax, we are also able to release tension from the mind through the way of releasing emotion. It was classically thought within Chinese Medicine that true transformation only happens when we let go of stored emotions. Through the release of emotions, which, as mentioned previously, are classed as harmful by-products of the mind, the Shen can remain calm and able to flow freely. By physically releasing tension, through Tui Na, for instance, the body will release emotional tension that has been stored within the physical tissues of the body, enabling us to feel more relaxed and our tissues to feel more mobile. Patients often feel calmer and lighter due to the body requiring less energy as it is not having to store such emotion.

Core principles of Tui Na

- Balancing Yin and Yang.

- Regulating the Zang Fu (internal organs).

- Opening and dredging the channels, and promoting the circulation of Qi, Blood and Body Fluids.

- Calming the Shen (mind) and releasing the emotions.

Benefits of Tui Na

When utilised and performed correctly, according to the principles of Tui Na and Chinese Medicine, Tui Na can have many benefits to the body. Although as practitioners of Tui Na we work to the principles of Chinese Medicine, it is also important to understand the benefits of Tui Na from a Western perspective. We want to explain to our patients how we are able to help them, without confusing them with terminology that they will not understand. The general benefits of Tui Na include realignment of the tissues and joints; acceleration of healing and reduction of the risk of reoccurring injuries; breaking down scar tissue and adhesions; and strengthening the immune system.

Realignment of the tissues and joints

One of the main principles and thought processes behind Tui Na is that, if the body is in alignment and everything is moving as it should, then the body should be able to heal and self-regulate. The body is an incredible organism that has the ability to self-regulate and self-repair, and as mentioned previously when discussing the regulation of the Zang Fu, when the channels are active and flowing smoothly, then the Qi and Blood can nourish the organs and the tissues, and the person will be healthy. However, sometimes the body struggles to heal and repair itself due to the damage or illness being too severe, or due to there being a physical misalignment that the body cannot correct by itself. What's more, the body can sometimes make a mess of healing itself, and make things worse. Using Tui Na, we can ensure that the tissues and joints of the body are properly aligned and sitting as they should be, encouraging and maintaining good posture, meaning that the body can then take care of itself in the best way possible. It is actually the body that does most of the healing, with the practitioner (through the use of Tui Na in this case) simply enabling and encouraging it to do so.

> ### The Qi Men (氣門)
>
> The *major joint spaces* within the skeletal system are sometimes referred to as the *Qi Men*, or *Qi Gates*. It is at these *'gates'* (spaces within the joints) that *Qi* and *Blood* can gather and are most likely to *stagnate*.

Within the Chinese Arts, the major joint spaces within the skeletal system are sometimes referred to as the Qi Men (氣門), or Qi Gates. It is at these 'gates' (spaces within the joints) that Qi and Blood can gather and are most likely to stagnate. Imagine a busy six-lane motorway bottle-necking to just a couple of lanes before opening up again. This is why most swellings and inflammatory conditions occur at the joints (including arthritis and even eczema). With Tui Na, we work on the body to either relax or strengthen the soft tissues in order to stabilise the joints, and also create space within the joints through techniques such as Ba Shen Fa (traction), to enable a smooth flow of Qi and Blood. This reduces the likelihood of stagnation of Qi and Blood within the Qi Men. It is also important that there is stability within the joints to ensure that they can transfer strength and maintain alignment. By aligning the tissues and joints of the body, we can ensure that there is balance within the soft tissues supporting the bone structure, and that the joints can operate as they should in a neutral position.

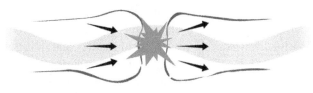

Qi flow through the Qi Men (氣門)

Acceleration of healing and reduction of the risk of reoccurring injuries

It is ultimately the function of our Wei Qi (衛氣) to heal injuries and damage done to the body tissues, and to restore and maintain regular functioning of the body. When we use Tui Na to treat our patients, we are essentially making their body's own healing mechanisms become more efficient. We are not adding anything to the body in terms of substance, but simply enabling the body to become more effective in what it does itself. By using Tui Na to open the channels, relax any tension and to realign the body (whether this be by realigning the bone structure or the Sinew channels), Qi and Blood will be able to flow unobstructed, and healing can occur in a quicker and smoother fashion. It is thought that the smoother and quicker healing occurs, the better the body can heal and return to its original state. It is unlikely that the body will ever repair entirely as good as new, although the closer we can get it to returning to its original state, the better the repair will be, and the less risk of an injury happening again at the same site due to weakness. When the body does not heal smoothly, there may be future complications with greater chance of bodily compensations, build-ups of scar tissues and adhesions, or simply weaker body and tissue structures.

Breaking down scar tissue and adhesions

As mentioned above, when the body attempts to heal itself, it may sometimes do so in a crude fashion that creates a build-up of scar tissue and adhesions. This is often unavoidable, as the body can never heal to a state that it was once originally. However, with the use of specific Tui Na techniques, we can locate and break down scar tissue and adhesions that may have appeared over time during the healing of previous or current injuries, and encourage the body to heal in a smoother fashion. Additionally, by relaxing and softening the surrounding tissues that have transformed due to compensation of any scar tissue or adhesions, the area will begin to relax and return to a more natural state that will allow better circulation. Although it is argued that actual scar tissue cannot be truly altered once it has developed, simply by transforming the surrounding tissues, patients will feel that the scar tissue has indeed been transformed, and circulation will improve.

Strengthening the immune system

From a Chinese Medicine perspective, it is our Wei Qi that governs our immunity. When our immune system becomes compromised, the lymphatic fluids become stagnated and more viscous. Essentially, when our Wei Qi becomes deficient, it lacks the motive force to help circulate the lymphatic fluids throughout the body, and it also lacks the warming function that helps to keep our vessels open. The vessels constrict and the flow of Blood and lymphatic fluid slows down. This further harms our immune system as it makes it more difficult to protect us against disease. Tui Na helps to keep the Qi, Blood and Body Fluids moving, whilst also activating and stimulating the Wei Qi. By mobilising the Qi, Blood and Body Fluids, the body can resist and fight off pathogens. Massage in general has also been shown to increase the number of lymphocytes within the body, which are a type of white blood cell that acts to protect the body from disease, again, by stimulating the Wei Qi and allowing the natural defence mechanisms of the body to take place.

Benefits of Tui Na

- Realignment of the tissues and joints.

- Acceleration of healing and reduction of the risk of reoccurring injuries.

- Breaking down scar tissue and adhesions.

- Strengthening the immune system.

Safe practice of Tui Na

The difference between a caution and a contraindication is that, when something is considered a caution, it can still be done, although under extreme care and attention. A thorough understanding of the condition and caution is a must for safe practice. A contraindication, on the other hand, is when something should not be done under any circumstances as there is danger of causing further damage to the patient. Above all, common sense is essential, and the saying 'when in doubt, leave it out' is highly important!

In order to establish cautions and contraindications, a full consultation is necessary. Unless a full consultation has been given, along with a detailed medical history, then everything should be considered a contraindication. Once a full consultation has been given, informed consent is needed before any physical contact is made. This is to make the patient aware of what will be happening during the treatment, and to ensure that they are happy for you to proceed. Patients are often in discomfort or pain, and Tui Na can at times be uncomfortable. This should be made clear before any treatment is given.

Safe practice of Tui Na

- Always take a full consultation including a detailed medical history.

- Before any physical contact with the patient, gain written informed consent.

- Only use suitable techniques or manipulations appropriate to the patient's age, constitution and condition.

Contraindications (Tui Na should *not* be given)

A contraindication means that treatment should *not* be done for one reason or another. It is usually due to the potential of more harm being caused to the patient. Not all contraindications mean that *no* treatment can be given, with some contraindications simply referring to specific areas of the body. In some cases, treatment can still be given to other parts of the body or adapted in nature. Key contraindications in the treatment of Tui Na can be found below:

- The patient does not want treatment (This may sound obvious, but is of the utmost importance.)

- At a bone fracture site during early stages.

- In an area of broken skin.

- During an acute skin eruption such as scabies, herpes, eczema or psoriasis (Tui Na should not be done in the area affected).

- In the presence of an infectious disease.

- If the patient has a severe cardiovascular or circulatory disorder, such as myocarditis, pericarditis, severe hypertension, deep vein thrombosis, an embolism or blood clot.

- If the patient experiences increased pain upon palpation.

Cautions (extreme care *must* be taken)

As mentioned above, a caution means that Tui Na can indeed be done, although extreme care must be taken. When deciding to perform some of the more complex or powerful techniques within Tui Na, it is always the case that the practitioner should think, 'is there a reason that I should not be doing this?' However, when there are cautions involved, it should be more of a case of, 'is there a reason that I need to be doing this?' Key cautions in the treatment of Tui Na can be found below:

- During pregnancy (it is contraindicated to use points SP-6, LI-4, BL-60, BL-67, GB-21, lower abdominal points below the naval and any points on the sacrum).

- In the presence of deformities or abnormalities.

- In the presence of swellings.

- If there is neuropathy.

- In the presence of cancer.*

- When the patient is taking certain medications such as steroids (long-term use) or blood thinners.

- When treating patients with internal diseases such as heart disease, cancer* or disease of the mind.

- When treating the weak, the very old or the young.

- When treating recent traumatic injuries.

---

* It is largely debated whether or not Tui Na (or any other massage therapy) can be done should the patient be suffering from a form of cancer. The best advice in cases like this is to first check with the patient's consultant oncologist. Written consent from the patient's consultant oncologist should be sought for peace of mind for both the practitioner and the patient.

Chapter 2

Approaches to Practice and Practitioner Development

Classically, the first introduction to Tui Na (or Chinese bodywork therapy) was through the training of a Martial Art. It was considered necessary to first understand a Martial Art in order to understand the body mechanics from an experiential way of learning. A Martial Art will demonstrate how the joints should move, how the weight should shift, and how the body can generate power through relaxation and body structure. This was considered necessary for understanding how to perform Tui Na techniques efficiently, understanding the natural alignments of the body for techniques such as bone setting and joint manipulations, and how the body should move for diagnostic purposes. If one could understand these concepts in relation to themselves, through Martial Arts for instance, it was thought that they could understand them from a patient's perspective.

It was also considered important to understand a self-cultivation system such as Nei Gong, Qi Gong or meditation. These practices would help to cultivate the practitioner and benefit them in understanding how to engage the Yi (意, intent), and apply the acts of Song (松, letting go) and Ting (聽, listening).

In modern practice, it is not considered 'mandatory' to engage in self-cultivation practices or understand a Martial Art (although these activities most certainly do help); however, the principles taken from certain Chinese Arts are still used for the development of Tui Na. The following should be taken into account whilst developing and practising your Tui Na:

- Duration of practice.

- Rice bags.

- Using both hands.

- Keeping warm.

- Breathing, relaxation and applying Song (松).

- Engaging the Yi (意) and using Ting (聽).

- Stretching and conditioning.

- Rooting.

- 'Understanding' rather than 'knowing'.

Approaches to practice

Duration of practice

Individual techniques should each be practised for long periods at a time. This is not only to become good at an individual technique, but also to build up the strength and structure required for clinical practice, and to build the necessary connections between the mind and body whilst performing the technique. To begin with, 5–10 minutes of each technique is enough, especially of the less complex techniques such as Na Fa and Mo Fa. More awkward techniques such as Gun Fa and Yi Zhi Chan Tui Fa should have more time spent on them, starting with 10–15 minutes and building up towards 30 minutes. Some schools suggest 30–40 hours of practice of each of the main 'simple' techniques before they should be used on a patient. This is why rice bags are ideal. Alternatively, whilst sitting, practice can be done for certain techniques on the thighs, giving you a feel for the technique as well as practising the movements.

A brief story about duration

During part of my training, I was developing a technique called Tan Bo Fa at a clinic in China. The particular teacher that I was with at the time was blind and did not speak English – I also did not speak Chinese! It was a tricky situation. Luckily I already knew the basics of most techniques from previous training, and I could recognise certain Chinese medical terminology, so when the teacher kept shouting "Bo, Bo, Bo", I knew that he wanted me to perform Tan Bo Fa on him (the techniques were performed on him so that he could tell if my technique was correct or not). I was made to do this, non-stop, for hours. My thumbs and hands were hurting and I just wanted to stop. Every time I went to take a break, again he would shout, "Bo, Bo, Bo". I kept going, and eventually my body could not take the discomfort any more because of the tension in my muscles and my hands, so I adjusted my technique to try and 'cheat' by avoiding use of those muscles so that they could rest. Just a few minutes after changing my technique, the teacher (in Chinese) said "Good", and made me move on to another technique. It turned out that by altering my technique to avoid the discomfort, I had changed to the correct way that the technique *should* have been performed. The duration and discomfort was something that I had to go through in order to understand the technique, and this understanding then transferred into other aspects of my Tui Na. Although, as a teacher of Tui Na, I teach and explain how to avoid poor technique to my students (rather than make them spend hours in discomfort to find out for themselves), I believe there is a great importance in going through this process in order to truly understand how to perform each technique. There should be a happy medium between being told how to do something, and being made to explore how to do something.

Rice bags

Classically, students would initially practice on a rice bag before moving on to patients or each other. This is still the case in many schools in China and also in some schools in the West. The use of rice bags is not to simply prevent injury to potential patients from an inexperienced student, but also to put more emphasis on the hand technique before the attention is spread elsewhere. When practising on a rice bag, the focus is almost entirely on the hand technique – how it moves, how it feels (to the practitioner), and how it looks and so on. Naturally, we are not concerned about how the rice bag is feeling! As soon as a technique is being applied to a body, some of the focus is drawn away from the technique and placed into the patient's body, with the student being mindful of how and what the patient is feeling. I personally think it is important to regularly practise on a rice bag, even once qualified, as this helps the practitioner to always improve on technique and make the minor adjustments that may not be noticed during a busy clinic.

Using both hands

Practice of both hands is important. With the varying contours of the human body, it is sometimes necessary to change hands when performing a technique in order to maintain posture, structure and power. Not only this, but if a practitioner always uses their dominant hand, they will become tired and overworked much quicker than if they were to use both hands, and the dominant hand would potentially suffer injury.

There are two ways that a student can develop using both hands. My personal preference when learning was to gain competence with my dominant hand initially, so then my less dominant hand had a point of reference, both visually and kinesthetically – not only did I know what the technique should look like, I also knew how it should *feel* to me as a practitioner. This enabled my less dominant hand to improve much quicker as it had another point of reference to go by. The other method is to simply spend equal time training each hand. Either way, it is essential to be fully competent with both hands in order to be adaptable to any situation such as awkward positioning or injury of one hand.

Keeping warm

Just like warming up is important to an athlete, it is important to warm up and keep warm before and during Tui Na. Many of my patients will comment that 'Tui Na must be quite the workout for you', and in some ways they are right, so we should treat it that way in order to work efficiently and without injury. When we are cold, our tissues contract; when we are warm, our tissues expand. The very nature of heat is to expand and to move, which is exactly what we want for the Qi and Blood when we are practising Tui Na. For a Tui Na practitioner, Qi and Blood circulation to the palms and finger tips is essential in order to increase sensitivity for diagnosis. Warmth is equally important to help with a full range of motion and free movement within the joints for when we are performing our hand techniques in order to prevent injury from 'wear and tear'. Besides, your patient will also appreciate warm hands rather than being shocked by cold hands!

Breathing, relaxation and applying Song (松, letting go)

As mentioned above in regards to keeping warm, it is essential that our tissues and joints are relaxed so that we maintain the full range of motion and free movement within the joint spaces, and maintain flexibility and space within the Sinew channels. This is essential in order for us to prevent injury to ourselves whilst performing the techniques used within Tui Na. In addition to keeping warm, another way to ensure relaxation of the tissues and joints is through our breathing and by applying Song (松). Song is essentially a form of release that comes about through the act of 'letting go' of any tension through the energetic body in order to help release tension stored within the consciousness or physical body – it is relaxation with structure. This is often done through correct posture and breathing techniques. It is an integral aspect of many of the Chinese Arts, and is necessary within Tui Na in order to maintain prolonged practice and the correct transfer of Qi, and entirely necessary in order to apply the act of Ting (聽), discussed later.

Within Chinese Medicine, it is held that the Lungs help to regulate and control the Liver, and it is the Liver that controls the sinews and tendons. When the tendons and sinews are tight, and the Liver is constrained, it is our Lungs (and therefore our breathing) that helps to regulate the Liver to enable the sinews and tendons to relax and release, thus allowing the Qi and Blood to flow more freely. This is why simply focusing on the act of Song and your breathing during times of stress can massively help with stress reduction, and why breathing exercises are so important within methods of relaxation.

Balancing Yin and Yang through the breath

There are many breathing techniques within Chinese Medicine that create specific movements within the body and help to regulate the vital substances. A simple method to help harmonise Yin and Yang within the body, creating a balance between relaxation and activation, is to gently breathe in for 4–5 seconds, hold your breath in for 4–5 seconds (tonifying Yang), gently breathe out for 4–5 seconds, and then hold your breath out for 4–5 seconds (nourishing Yin). Repeat this process for around 5 minutes. It is also important that each transition between the stages of breath are smooth and not forced (for example, after breathing in, do not forcefully hold your breath then suddenly let it out). By doing this, we are essentially increasing the level of oxygen within the body that helps with activation of the tissues, whilst also increasing the level of carbon dioxide that causes vasodilation of the blood vessels, therefore creating warmth, relaxation and better circulation.

In addition to the breath and the act of Song greatly helping to relax the sinews and tendons, and releasing tension within the joints, breathing also helps to descend the Qi for us to remain rooted and grounded, as it is a function of the Lungs to descend the Qi to the lower parts of the body. This is important due to the fact that being well grounded allows for better transfer of power, and enables the practitioner to draw power from the ground and through their body structure rather than generating power with the tendons and muscles. An excellent book that covers Song breathing is *A Comprehensive Guide to Daoist Nei Gong*, by Damo Mitchell.

Engaging the Yi (意, intent) and using Ting (聽, listening)

In Chinese Medicine, the Yi (意) is the psychological aspect related to the Spleen, and is likened in Western medicine to our intellect, cognitive ability and intent. Some may also refer to it as our ability to 'focus'. As mentioned in the beginning of this section, it is massively important that a Tui Na practitioner works with intent rather than simply and mindlessly applying techniques to a patient. The reason Tui Na is called 'pushing and grasping' is because each technique performed should encompass either of these two movements of Qi. This should be done both on a physical level and on a psychological level, which can be directed by our Yi.

There is a famous Chinese saying, 'Where the Yi goes, the Qi follows'. I find both within my own practice, and when my students are practising, that there is a huge difference in the quality and effectiveness of a technique whether the mind/intent is in the patient, in the hand performing the technique (as it often is at the beginning of study), or somewhere else altogether (for example, thinking about what you are going to have for dinner that evening). On a physical level, changing the type and level of intent will subconsciously cause many minor adjustments in the tissues of the practitioner, all of which add up and can completely change the quality and effectiveness of the technique. It is important that we put our mind into the body of the patient and have the intent on what our desired effect is. Even if our mind is in the hand that is performing the technique or at the point of contact between the hand and patient, it is not good enough, as this will cause stagnation of Qi within the hand and the Qi will not flow properly into the patient.

Engaging the Yi (意)

Within the Chinese Arts it is thought to be important to 'feed' and 'train' the Yi (意) with knowledge of the subject, and therefore to allow the Yi to develop and grow in a certain way in order to gain greater focus and intent whilst performing the physical aspect of the specific art.

Knowing the importance of engaging and training the Yi in regards to technique quality and effectiveness also demonstrates the importance of understanding the theories and principles that underpin any physical practice. Within the Chinese Arts it is thought to be important to 'feed' and 'train' the Yi with knowledge of the subject, and therefore to allow the Yi to develop and grow in a certain way in order to gain greater focus and intent whilst performing the physical aspect of the specific art. This is why it is important to have thorough understanding of the theoretical aspect of any practice in addition to the practical aspect.

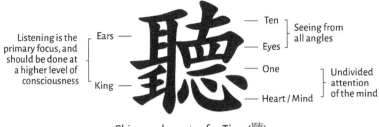

Listening is the primary focus, and should be done at a higher level of consciousness — Ears — King — Ten — Eyes — Seeing from all angles — One — Heart / Mind — Undivided attention of the mind

Chinese character for Ting (聽)

Within the Chinese Arts, the term 'Ting' (聽) is most commonly translated as 'listening', and refers to a state of awareness and mindfulness that should always be present during our practice. It is essentially the act of being fully engaged in what we are doing at a depth that involves the undivided attention of the conscious mind in addition to using the ears, eyes and touch to 'listen'. The written Chinese character, shown above, details quite nicely the term 'Ting' and what the act of 'listening' requires.

To the left of the character, we have the symbol for 'Ear' (耳) situated above and embracing the symbol for 'King' or 'Monarch' (王). This part of the character tells us that the character has the overall meaning of 'listening', with the King symbol being used to tell us that the act of listening is the primary focus. It is necessary to note here that it is the act of listening rather than the act of hearing that is important, and not literally the use of the ears. The King, often referred to as the Monarch, also represents a hierarchy in terms of our consciousness (which is why the Heart is often termed the 'Monarch' in the Chinese Arts). This again indicates that Ting should be done at a depth of consciousness that engages the Shen rather than idly listening.

Situated at the top right of the character are the symbols for 'Ten' (十) and 'Eyes' (目). These two characters together represent the ability to view something from many angles and seeing it as a whole, with Ten being the number of completion. Similarly to what was mentioned above with the ears, it is necessary to understand that it is the act of looking rather than the act of seeing that is important, and not literally the use of the eyes.

The bottom right of the character consists of the symbols for 'One' (一) situated over the symbol for the Heart/Mind (心). Together, these characters mean one mind, otherwise referred to as our undivided attention. It is this level and depth of awareness that is required during the act of Ting, in that we should apply our full focus and attention to the situation at hand.

When practising Tui Na, we expand our awareness through the act of Ting throughout our entire body as well as into the patient's body. It is this quality of awareness that first of all allows our body to create the correct shapes, structures and postures, and then allows us to establish a correct diagnosis, and to perform the correct technique at the correct depth.

The act of Ting (聽)

The act of Ting (聽, listening) allows us to have a quality of awareness that helps us to establish a correct diagnosis, and to perform the correct technique at the correct depth.

Stretching and conditioning

As with any physical activity, the body of the practitioner needs to achieve and maintain a certain state of conditioning in order to efficiently and effectively deliver treatment. Although we do not require strength for Tui Na in the form of 'muscular power', we do, of course, require the strength and conditioning of the body's tissues in order to perform techniques correctly and powerfully (if needed) for potentially long periods of time.

Stretching opens the joints and enables relaxation of the tissues in order for Qi and Blood to flow freely through the channels, and to allow the Sinew channels (Jing Jin) to activate and deactivate when necessary in order for the practitioner to deliver power, yet stay relaxed enough to make it through multiple treatments without tiring. Staying relaxed is vital in order to transmit Qi through the channels.

Conditioning gives strength and endurance to the practitioner. Even though there is a lot of emphasis on relaxation and 'empty' hand techniques, it is necessary to build strength in order to have the power to achieve the desired effects of certain techniques.

Rooting

When carrying out a Tui Na treatment, it is essential that the practitioner stays rooted and allows the power of each technique to be transferred *through* the practitioner's body rather than be *produced by* the body. Good rooting is achieved through correct posture, relaxation and also intent. Essentially, the bone structure should be aligned to stay strong and upright, with the muscles relaxed just enough to support yet 'hang' from the bones.

When a student or practitioner is new to Tui Na, they may find that their body aches in places such as the wrists, arms and shoulders, neck, and even the lower back. This is mostly due to misalignment of the body because correct posture and technique has not yet developed, and the power is being generated from the muscles and tendons rather than through structure and good technique. Once the student or practitioner becomes more efficient at both technique and at transferring power from the ground and through body structure, they will notice that only the soles of the feet will ache due to the force being transferred to and from the ground – the feet may feel like they would do as if there had been a heavy weight bearing downwards on the body. Intent is also an important part of this transfer of power, and should be directed both downwards towards the ground, and outwards towards the patient.

Maintaining correct posture whilst practising Tui Na is absolutely crucial – not just for practitioner safeguarding and prevention of injury, but also for correct technique and power delivery. Even the slightest deviation in posture can change the whole nature of a technique and alter the direction of power. This is so often missed within teachings of Tui Na, with most emphasis being placed on hand or even arm techniques. Some teachers may even go as far as correcting the alignment of the upper posture. However, something as small as the back foot being slightly pointed in the wrong direction, or even the knees not being relaxed enough, can have a huge impact on the positioning of the hand. This is not really something that can be taught or learned from a book, as it takes many minor adjustments from a qualified teacher to help the student to 'sit' comfortably in their posture, with as little tension as possible. The posture also changes throughout the many positions that we assume throughout treatment whilst moving around the treatment couch. Once it becomes second nature to keep the body in an open, relaxed, yet aligned posture, and that it feels wrong when the body is not positioned in this way, we can be a little more loose with these posture guidelines as the body knows how to maintain correct posture, even in awkward positions. We can then compromise our posture, for example, by assuming seated positions or awkward standing positions, because we have essentially trained the lines of power delivery. Of course, once the student has embodied the principles of posture and structure, these rules and principles can be broken. This can be done because the student will know *how* to break them, in addition to knowing when and when not to break them. However, whilst first learning the basic shapes of Tui Na, it is important to stick to the following general guidelines as this helps to develop the correct structures and lines for power delivery. Although there are too many variables in Tui Na body positioning to cover in writing, some key principles that should be taken into consideration within *any* position are as follows:

- When performing Tui Na, the upper body should always be upright, or in line with the back leg, if needing to lean forward. This prevents tension stagnating at the lower back, and creates a transfer of power from the ground and through to the arms rather than being generated from the upper body. The feet and knees should be pointing in the same direction as the hips, which should have a strong connection to the shoulders and also point in the same direction. This may appear like a Martial Arts stance, which it is, and uses the same principles to deliver power through structure and relaxation. The stance can be long if the treatment couch is low, or the stance can be short if the technique is performed high.

- The arms should never cross the body. For example, if I am standing to the right of my patient, and using Gun Fa *down* the right side of the body, I would use my left hand. Using my right hand would cause me to cross my body unless I was using it to go *up* the patient's body. Crossing the body is poor practice as it closes the gates of Qi that travel through the shoulder into the arm, especially within the arm Yin channels. It is important that we keep these open to allow smoother flow of Qi and Blood. Some schools say that you should always be able to fit a fist just below the armpit, as this region is vital for the transferal of power.

- When using techniques such as Rou Fa, Tui Fa or Gun Fa with the forearm, it is also important that the forearm is in a neutral position, in that the radius and ulna do not pronate or supinate. This provides slightly more strength within the Sinew channels, better flow of Qi, and also presents a better edge of the ulna bone whilst performing the massage techniques. The upper arm should also not be collapsed, and should have a strong angle away from the body. This helps to protect the shoulder and prevent any wrongful direction of force.

- Lastly, it is quite common for new students to 'bob' up and down whilst performing certain rhythmical techniques. This is poor practice, and causes the power to be consumed before it is transferred into the patient. This also disrupts the rooting of the practitioner and disperses the Yi. The stance should be strong, focused and grounded. Movement should be fluid, and only necessary movement should be made with only the necessary tissues engaged.

'Understanding' rather than 'knowing'

Emphasis on the main 'simple' techniques/manipulations is fundamental before going on to practise 'complex' techniques/manipulations. I am a huge believer in saying that the difference between 'knowing how to perform' a technique and 'understanding and internalising' a technique is *massive*. A practitioner can only understand the true energy or nature of a technique once they have spent many hours practising, feeling and observing a technique. This is how a technique becomes a *skill* (功, Gong) rather than a *method* (法, Fa). Many of the complex techniques have also developed from simple hand techniques. Refraining from jumping ahead is sometimes tough but essential in becoming a solid Tui Na practitioner.

The nine therapeutic methods of Tui Na (Jiu Fa, 九法)

The nine therapeutic methods of Tui Na (Jiu Fa, 九法) are based on the eight therapeutic methods (Ba Fa, 八法) that were originally discussed within *Huang Di Nei Jing Su Wen* that underpin the main therapeutic principles of Acupuncture and Chinese Herbal Medicine. Chapter 74 of the *Su Wen* notes that:

> Treatment principles consist of warming to dispel cold, cooling to clear heat, dispersing to remove congestion, purging to eliminate build up, catharsis to dispel water (Phlegm), lubricating to moisten dryness, fortifying to strengthen deficiency, decelerating to arrest acute progression, invigorating to accelerate flow, inducing vomiting to expel food or phlegm, calming to tranquilise anxiety, and softening to dissolve mass.

These 12 methods have since been combined into the eight therapeutic methods of Chinese Medicine based on their therapeutic actions, and have again since been adapted for use within Tui Na with the addition of the dredging method. These nine methods are: *tonifying, reducing, dredging, sweating, dissipating, harmonising, warming, clearing* and *emesis*.

In addition to choosing techniques based on their actions and indications that are discussed in Section 3, techniques would be used in accordance with the nine therapeutic methods, which would be guided by the treatment principles. For example, within the foundation theories of Chinese Medicine it is held that when there is deficiency, one should tonify; when there is excess, one should reduce; when there is heat, one should clear heat; when there is cold, one should warm; when there is stagnation, one should resolve and so on. These therapeutic principles can be carried by a number of methods and by using a number of the simple techniques. It is important to understand the actions and indications of each therapeutic method, as it is indeed possible to choose the wrong technique and wrong therapeutic method, therefore making the patient worse. Tui Na is, of course, a medical intervention, and as with any other medical intervention, care should be given.

In modern practice, certain therapeutic principles such as inducing vomiting (emesis) are no longer used. However, it is useful to understand the nine methods in order to gain a fuller understanding of Tui Na and how it was used as a whole medical system. It is also uncommon to use a single therapeutic method. Instead, it is more practical to combine therapeutic methods as diseases in modern times are often complex and often in a state of flux. The nine therapeutic methods of Tui Na are as follows.

补法 Bu Fa (tonifying)

'Bu' means to tonify, strengthen or reinforce. Along with Xie Fa (reducing), it is one of the main therapeutic methods used within Chinese Medicine. How to adapt techniques in order to tonify will be discussed in greater detail below.

It should be noted that strong tonifying techniques should be used with caution when the patient is suffering from external Wind-Heat or Wind-Cold presenting as flu-like symptoms, as this can cause external pathogens to travel deeper into the body and exacerbate the condition.

泻法 Xie Fa (reducing)

'Xie Fa' means to reduce or to drain. This is used in order to reduce tension, or when there are any signs of excess in any way. Along with Bu Fa, it is one of the main therapeutic methods used within Chinese Medicine. How to adapt techniques in order to reduce will be discussed in more detail below.

疏浚法 Shu Jun Fa (dredging)

Dredging refers to the clearing of a channel, and in some cases, a joint. As the Jing Luo system of the body is considered to be like a network of rivers and pathways, the term 'dredging' is used in the same way as 'dredging a river bed'. Dredging, in the same way as physically dredging a river, is used in order to clear a channel and remove any unwanted blockages, pathogens or 'debris' from a channel and/or joint. As the saying goes in Chinese Medicine, 'wherever there is pain, there is a blockage'. It is important to ensure that the channels and joints are free from any blockages and pathogens in order to ensure the Qi and Blood can flow smoothly along a channel and through the joints. Tui Na is perhaps the most effective method of treatment in regards to physically dredging the channels out of the various modalities of Chinese Medicine (including Acupuncture, Herbal Medicine and Qi Gong). This will help to reduce and prevent pain, numbness, swelling and also Blood stasis. Dredging is one of the most commonly used therapeutic methods in Tui Na and is often used in conjunction with another method such as opening the channels, warming the channels or clearing the channels. Certain techniques such as Tui Fa are specifically used to dredge the channels, whereas techniques such as Ba Shen Fa are used to dredge a joint.

汗法 Han Fa (sweating)

The sweating method, also known as diaphoresis, causes the pores to open in order to release the body's exterior and to primarily regulate the Lung Qi. It is mainly used in the treatment of exterior conditions and for patients who have been invaded by either Wind-Cold or Wind-Heat, where it is needed to expel the excess pathogens from their exterior through sweating. With Tui Na, techniques such as An Fa and Yi Zhi Chan can be used on key points such as GB-20 (Feng Chi), DU-16 (Feng Fu), LI-4 (He Gu), and SJ-5 (Wai Guan) in order to stimulate the body's healing response to external Wind. Strong stimulation of these points are known to induce sweating. Alternatively, quick and gentle stimulation of the Tai Yang channels through techniques such as Na Fa, Ca Fa and Pai Fa can also cause the body to induce sweating and help to release external pathogens.

The sweating method should be avoided with deficiency-type syndromes where the patient is already sweating, and should only be used for short periods of time so as to avoid injuring the Yin. *It should also be noted that in cases of Blood deficiency, sweating could make the condition worse, as Blood and Body Fluids are of the same origin, and sweat is the fluid of the Heart.*

消散法 Xiao San Fa (dissipating)

The dissipating method refers to the dispersal and movement of stagnations and accumulations. Dissipating stagnations and masses within the superficial layers of the body or the channels may be done with the use of Yi Zhi Chan Tui Fa. For example, for fullness and stagnation in the sinuses causing headache, in practice I may use Yi Zhi Chan Tui Fa applied to EX-M-HN-3 (Yin Tang), which can help to resolve the stagnation and open up the channels. Dissipating masses on a deeper level may be done with techniques such as Zhen Fa. For instance, constipation due to stagnation of the Large Intestine may be treated by Zhen Fa applied to the lower abdomen to dissipate and break down masses to encourage bowel movement.

和法 He Fa (harmonising)

Within modern Chinese Medicine, the term 'harmonising' is often used non-specifically, for example, to 'harmonise the Liver', or to 'harmonise menstruation'. However, its 'true' meaning is to bring two separate things into balance and return their functional relationship to a natural state, for example, to 'harmonise the Heart and Kidneys'. In Tui Na, and especially within the treatment of musculoskeletal conditions, this may mean to bring harmony to the relationship between opposing muscle groups, or the relationship between tension and relaxation. In Acupuncture or Herbal Medicine, it is commonly used in the treatment of Shao Yang syndrome, where it is important to both expel pathogens from the exterior whilst also tonifying the interior. Essentially, the harmonising method would be used in complex cases where there is both excess and deficiency, for instance.

In the practice of Tui Na, the harmonising method is most commonly used in order to regulate the flow of Qi and Blood (and therefore circulation), restoring balance between the Sinew channels, and also returning normal function to specific bodily functions such as the menstrual cycle. Techniques would usually be soft and continuous, with a focus on versatile techniques such as Mo Fa, Gun Fa and Rou Fa. In regards to treating internal conditions through the use of Tui Na, the harmonising method would make use of key acupoints, such as using Yi Zhi Chan on SP-8 (Di Ji) that would be used to 'harmonise the menses', which ultimately means to return normality and regularity to the menstrual cycle.

温法 Wen Fa (warming)

The warming therapeutic method is generally used with deficient conditions where Cold is present, or when there is an excess of the Cold pathogen within the channels. The warming method may also be applied along with the dissipating method in order to remove stagnation by causing the channels to expand and open and invigorating the flow of Qi and Blood.

In my practice, I would use techniques such as Mo Fa or Ca Fa to generate heat in a specific area, such as the lower lumbar on points such as DU-4 (Ming Men) or the abdomen on points such as R-12 (Zhong Wan). The difference between deficiency Cold or excess Cold would be to use gentle and slow manipulations or vigorous and quick manipulations respectively.

清法 Qing Fa (clearing)

The clearing method involves using certain techniques to clear Heat from the body. Heat as a pathogen can occur at different levels within the body, including within the channels, within the Blood and within the organs. When using Tui Na techniques to clear Heat, we do so by directing Yang Qi downwards and also by nourishing Yin. We can also use techniques to open up the channels, such as stimulating the Jing Well or Back Shu points to clear Heat from the channels.

In addition to stimulating certain points in order to clear Heat, such as the Jing Well (channel Heat) or Back Shu (organ Heat), in my practice I use techniques such as Tui Fa downwards along the Du channel, therefore sedating Yang Qi within the channels. When treating cases of Heat due to Yin deficiency, I may use techniques such as Rou Fa or Yi Zhi Chan Tui Fa on BL-23 (Shen Shu), to nourish the Kidneys to support Yin.

吐法 Tu Fa (emesis)

Emesis is the method of inducing the vomiting reflex to purge the stomach of pathogens. This method of treatment is not used so much in modern practice, and not a method I have ever used on a patient within my own practice (for quite obvious reasons!). It may, however, be a method that you need to use on yourself, as purging pathogens from the stomach can help to speed up the recovery of sickness bugs or poisoning, or recovery from severe food retention.

The easiest method to induce vomiting is to get the patient to put their own fingers into their throat. Other ways to induce vomiting would be to press on the lower abdomen with two fingers or the palm root just above the umbilicus, and press inward and upward towards R-12 (Zhong Wan). This method is particularly useful to expel severe food retention in the stomach.

The nine therapeutic methods of Tui Na (Jiu Fa, 九法)

− Tonifying	− Reducing	− Dredging
− Sweating	− Dissipating	− Harmonising
− Warming	− Clearing	− Emesis

Tonifying (Bu, 补) and reducing (Xie, 泻) methods using Tui Na

The terms 'tonifying' and 'reducing' are used a lot within Chinese Medicine, and are the foundation of most treatments. Essentially, when something is not there that should be, such as Qi or Blood, or when something is weaker than it should be, then we tonify or strengthen. If something is there that shouldn't be, such as stagnation or pathogens, then we reduce and purge the excess pathogenic factors. The difference between deficient and excess conditions, especially in regards to the Sinew channels, will be discussed in more depth within Section 2.

Within Tui Na, tonifying and reducing can be done by adapting the basic techniques and manipulations, such as altering the strength of the technique, the direction of the technique and the direction that it is applied along the channels. Whenever we perform Tui Na, we are effectively altering the state of Qi and Blood within the tissues, which then have an impact on the rest of the body. The following are ways that techniques can be adapted in order to either tonify or reduce.

Tonify or reduce using pressure

When applying pressure and strength to various Tui Na techniques, such as Rou Fa (kneading), it is generally accepted that lighter pressure with milder stimulation is more tonifying and nourishing, whereas heavier pressure with stronger stimulation is more reducing. When applying lighter pressure, techniques should be done for longer periods of time to stimulate growth and reinforcement. To tonify is to nourish, to generate and to nurture. When applying stronger and heavier pressure, techniques should be done for shorter periods of time to prevent damage and soreness or to prevent too much depletion.

For example, when a patient presents with a deficient condition such as a cough and asthma due to Lung Qi deficiency, I may use light techniques such as Mo Fa (circular rubbing) and Rou Fa (kneading) on the upper back to help nourish the Lungs, with gentle and prolonged stimulation of Fei Shu (BL-13), Ding Chuan (M-BW-1), Yun Men (LU-2) and Qi Hai (R-6). Should a patient present with an excess condition such as headache due to neck pain and muscle spasm, I would use strong and heavy pressure on Feng Chi (GB-20), Jian Jing (GB-21) and Jian Wai Shu (SI-14) and so on for shorter periods of time. This would help to reduce the tension and stagnation, and allow Qi and Blood to flow freely in and out of the head. The difference between stronger and milder stimulation will differ from patient to patient and will depend on the patient's age and constitution.

Tonify or reduce using rotation

A number of techniques and manipulations within Tui Na use rotation. When using the rotating direction to tonify or reduce, there are a couple of contradicting opinions as to which direction does what. With Tui Na, the direction is the same as Acupuncture, in that with your right hand it is considered to be clockwise for tonifying or anti-clockwise for reducing. It would be the opposite if you were to use your left hand. This is due to the movement of Qi within our bodies, and the way it moves as we move. Another way to think of this would be to rotate in the direction of the thumb to tonify, or against the thumb to reduce.

Tonify or reduce using channel direction

Within the *Su Wen*, it discusses tonifying and reducing methods in regards to the direction of flow within the Primary channels. That is, to tonify you would go with the channel, and to reduce you would go against the channel (the Primary channels flow both to and from the body, depending on which channel it is). This is indeed the case when using the Primary channels for treatment of the interior, for instance; however, when treating the exterior of the body, it is slightly different. When treating external conditions, we primarily work with the Sinew channels. As discussed later, each Sinew channel begins on the fingers or the toes at the Jing Well points, and then flows *towards* the body. This means that if we are to tonify the Sinew channels, we treat towards the body, whereas if we need to reduce the Sinew channel(s), we would treat away from the body and towards the fingers and/or toes.

Tonifying and reducing

When using *channel direction* to *tonify* or *reduce*, the difference between *Primary* channels and *Sinew* channels is an important differentiation to make because *treatment principles* will be different.

When using Tui Na to influence the Primary channels, we would treat according to the description within the classic text *Su Wen*, which is to tonify by treating in the direction of flow, or to reduce by treating against the direction of flow. This differs from channel to channel. All Yin channels of the body flow upwards from the feet to the body, and from the body down to the hands. All Yang channels flow upwards from the hands to the head, and from the head downwards to the feet. Therefore, tonifying the Yin channels would require techniques to be performed up the legs and outwards towards the hands, whereas tonifying the Yang channels would require techniques to be performed up the arms and down towards the feet. Reducing methods would be vice versa.

Type	Tonifying/reducing	Method
Pressure	Tonifying	Lighter pressure with milder stimulation for longer periods
	Reducing	Heavier pressure with stronger stimulation for shorter periods
Rotation direction	Tonifying	Rotating clockwise with your right hand, anti-clockwise with your left hand
	Reducing	Rotating anti-clockwise with your right hand, clockwise with your left hand
Channel direction	Tonifying	With the flow of the Sinew channels (towards the body)
	Reducing	Against the flow of the Sinew channels

Patient after-care

Tui Na can create a lot of changes within the body, some more noticeable than others, and it is always a good idea to explain to the patient what may happen over the next few hours and days following a treatment. This helps to put the patient's mind at ease should any 'negatively perceived' effects arise…

Effects after treatment

After receiving Tui Na, it is quite common for the patient to feel some soreness or tenderness. The patient may also feel a little energetically drained and lightheaded. It is important to warn the patient beforehand that this is quite normal and the lightheadedness should disappear after only a few minutes, and the discomfort should last only 24–48 hours or so. This can be worse if the patient had a lot of blockages or stagnation within the channels that have now been resolved. Below is an explanation of commonly seen reactions to treatment, and these are all reactions that the body makes when being transformed from one 'state' to another.

Soreness

Once the Sinew channels have been worked on quite strongly, the channels expand and contract whilst finding a comfortable position in which to settle down. This can cause discomfort within the joints and channels until they manage to find a comfortable position, which can take a couple of days.

When the patient is receiving treatment, especially in the case of excess conditions, practitioners are generally breaking tissue down. This is in order for the body to repair correctly. The patient does not get better whilst on the treatment couch; they will begin to heal over the days following the treatment. It is during the resting period after treatment that the patient will recover. Because the Sinew channels have been worked and realigned, the body feels sore as it repairs any tissues that have been broken down by directing the body's Wei Qi to the area. The Wei Qi collects at the site of injury and at the areas that have been worked on, creating minor swelling as the sinews begin to heal. The discomfort arises from the mild stagnation that is temporarily caused by the accumulation of Wei Qi and swelling. This is a perfectly normal reaction, and one that is necessary to the recovery process, and generally lasts only 24–48 hours or so.

Lightheadedness
The reason a patient may feel lightheaded or 'spaced out' after treatment is because the channel (Jing Luo) system has been stimulated, often increasing the circulation of Yang Qi throughout the body, now with less restriction. This fresh circulation of Qi can cause the body to relax and also feel lightheaded until the body is able to regulate itself and 'normalise'.

Tiredness
Occasionally the patient may feel tired for some time following a Tui Na treatment. This may last for just a few minutes or for the rest of the day, until the patient goes to bed. The reason that the patient feels tired is most likely because the energy system, primarily the Wei Qi, has been stimulated and gone into a state of healing. Tui Na essentially activates and accelerates the mechanism of healing, and if the patient has any underlying deficiencies or weaknesses, this can make them feel tired as their Qi is now being directed elsewhere rather than performing the basic actions of functioning. Although this is somewhat expected, in order to try to avoid any excessive tiredness, it is important to treat according to the constitution of the patient. If the patient is already weak, and a strong treatment is given for a longer period of time, it is likely that the patient will feel fatigued. This may have an opposite effect on the condition as the patient will not have the energy to respond to treatment.

After-care advice
In addition to warning the patient of any side effects that may occur after treatment, it is also good practice to give them advice that will help them to recover quicker. Patients do not get better during the one hour or so inside the treatment room, but during the time between treatments. Rather than us, as practitioners, doing all of the work, it is always much easier to teach and empower the patient to take their health into their own hands. Much like giving diet advice when prescribing herbs, giving your patient

after-care advice to do between Tui Na treatments will ensure that they improve much quicker than just relying on the one hour or so of treatment per week.

Dao Yin (導引) exercises

Dao Yin (導引) means to lead and to guide. Dao Yin exercises can be used to open up the joints, release the Sinew channels and, when more advanced, can be used to purge the channels of pathogens that have accumulated within the Sinew channels. It is important to keep exercises simple so that the patient is more likely to comply and perform the prescribed exercises on a regular basis. It is too common that patients are given multiple complex exercises, and this is more likely to put the patient off from doing the exercises that may be necessary in speeding up recovery. For some examples of Dao Yin exercises, see *Heavenly Streams* by Damo Mitchell (Singing Dragon) and *The Four Dragons* by Damo Mitchell (Singing Dragon).

External liniments, oils and balms

The use of liniments, oils and balms is excellent to help recovery in between Tui Na treatments. Depending on the requirement, there are many to choose from, and advice should be given to the patient on how to apply them and how often. There are a number of books that are very useful in regards to which medical liniments, oils or balms should be used for what, one well known book being *Tooth from the Tiger's Mouth* by Tom Bisio. For the sake of not 'reinventing the wheel', I suggest that you pick up this book for a good read on external liniments, oils and balms, and also how you can make them yourself. Below is a brief summary of some more common liniments, oils and balms.

External liniments, oils and balms	
Tiger Balm	Tiger Balm comes in two varieties, red or white. The red one is the more useful of the two. It contains a number of warming (with some cooling) herbs that help to open the channels and repair damaged tissues. Although it is very warming, especially at the Wei level, it is generally okay to use on acutely inflamed injuries. This is because the herbs that Tiger Balm contains are very powerfully moving, and can strongly aid in the healing process without making the inflammation worse, although to be on the safe side, I usually advise not using Tiger Balm until day two or three of an injury – it should be fine to use after that. Generally the white one is not quite as strong as the red one, and slightly less warming.
Wood Lock Oil	Wood Lock Oil is a famous brand of Huo Luo You, which basically means 'activate channel oil'. Wood Lock Oil should be used on areas of discomfort in order to open the channels and to enable a flow of Qi and Blood and to reduce pain whilst encouraging healing. It is similar to the way Tiger Balm works, although it is stronger and can spread further due to it being an oil rather than a balm.
Feng You Jing	Feng You Jing is a green, cooling oil that is very good for use on specific acupoints when a cooling effect is necessary. It can be used on specific acupoints at the beginning of treatment so that they are cooled and stimulated during the Tui Na treatment. Alternatively, it can be given to the patient to apply to specific points on a daily basis to help cool the channels. I have found it to be particularly useful for temporary relief of rheumatoid arthritis, if used correctly.

Feng Shi You	Feng Shi You is essentially the opposite of Feng You Jing, and can be used to treat Cold pathogens in the channels. Again, not much is needed and just a drop or two on specific acupoints is very useful before or in between treatments.
Dit Da Jow/Die Da Yao	Roughly translated as 'hit fall wine', this is an alcohol liniment that is used within many Martial Arts schools, all of which will have their own formula (probably 'better than any other out there!'). Dit Da Jow is a herbal decoction containing around 20–30 different herbs, most of which encourage healing, repair and strengthen tendons and bones, and cool and move Blood to resolve Qi and Blood stasis. Although it may not feel as strong, a good Dit Da Jow will be stronger and penetrate deeper than any of the above liniments, oils or balms.
Zheng Gu Shui	Zheng Gu Shui directly translates as 'repair bone liquid'; however, it is also used to repair tendons and deep tissue damage. The term 'Gu', or 'bone', simply refers to its ability to treat at the deepest layer. Zheng Gu Shui is essentially a commercial version of Dit Da Jow, discussed above.

Ice versus heat

Within the field of physical bodywork therapy, there has been (and still is) a lot of advice regarding the application of ice and/or heat to an injury. Patients often get told conflicting information from different therapists, and rightly become frustrated as they are none the wiser about how to care for their injury. In this situation I will explain my advised choice and the reasons for my choice, and then if patients are still frustrated, I suggest they do what they feel is better for them.

I find one of the key issues is the household term R.I.C.E – Rest, Ice, Compression, Elevation. I agree with the R.C.E, but as a Chinese Medicine practitioner I do not believe that ice is the answer. However, because this acronym has been around for many decades, it is at the front of people's minds, so they reach for the bag of peas as soon as any kind of injury occurs, and they continue to use it for days.

Within Chinese Medicine there is a saying, 'ice is for dead people'. A bit extreme, perhaps! Ultimately, from a Chinese Medicine point of view, the extreme Cold Qi that penetrates the body from the application of ice causes constriction and tension within the local tissues and vessels, thus causing a restriction of Qi, Blood and Body Fluids. What's more is that the Cold Qi causes the contractive and inward movement of the Wei Qi, which has accumulated in the area (causing swelling and warmth) in order to heal the Sinew channels from injury. Due to this restriction and inward movement caused by extreme cold, the healing mechanism of Wei Qi is slowed down. Some patients may not mind that the healing is slower because they are not pro athletes or needing to get back on their feet so quickly; however, it is not just the duration we are concerned about. Slow healing creates 'rough' healing, as opposed to quick healing that creates 'smooth' healing. When an injury heals slowly, there is more chance that the injury can transmit to surrounding channels or areas, and for things to go wrong and deformities to develop in the long term, such as greater scar tissue build-up or long-term deformities to the bone structure. The ideal environment for the Wei Qi to heal an injury is for there to be gentle mobilisation of the area, suitable rest and appropriate treatment.

The reason we may need ice is when there is a possibility of haemorrhage. This is because ice can restrict the blood vessels to stop the internal bleeding. Even then, in my opinion, it is still risky, as once you remove the ice, the body will attempt to self-regulate by increasing the blood supply to the area to warm it up. Ice also numbs the area, creating temporary pain relief. This is enough to make people want to use it in the first place, when there is an acute injury.

As soon as an injury is older than a couple of days, there is definitely no need for ice. Many practitioners use ice to numb an area and reduce pain and inflammation temporarily, with no regard to how it is affecting the patient in the long run.

Chapter 3

The Sinew Channels (Jing Jin, 经筋)

Within Chinese Medicine, or many of the Chinese Arts for that matter, the anatomy and physiology of the body (and the way that it moves) are not viewed in the same way they are is in modern Western medicine. In regards to the physical aspects of the musculoskeletal system, for example, which is thought to comprise many isolated muscles, tendons and other connective tissues, the Chinese Medicine view on this would be a series of interconnected channels, structures and systems. The concept of these are really the cornerstone throughout all modalities of Chinese Medicine and indeed, the Chinese Arts, with an understanding of the Sinew channels being arguably the most important aspect of understanding any type of bodywork following Chinese Medicine. Without understanding these Chinese Medicine principles, we are not really practising Tui Na, but just a generic form of physical therapy. Techniques do not make the therapy; it is the core foundations and principles that make the therapy.

An introduction to the Sinew channels can be found in the Chinese Medicine classic text *Nei Jing Su Wen*, and the trajectories and dysfunctions are discussed in more detail in Chapter 13 of the *Ling Shu*. One of the most important things to keep in mind as a student of Tui Na, and especially for those who have previously studied Acupuncture or other aspects of Chinese Medicine, is to avoid applying the same theory of the Primary channels to the Sinew channels. The mistake that people make in Tui Na when focusing on the Primary channels of Chinese Medicine theory rather than the Sinew channels is that they miss out vital parts of the channel and vital relationships between parts of the body (that are both diagnostic and relevant to treatment prescriptions), and misunderstand the behaviour and functions of Qi and Blood within the channels. These are very common mistakes, with many Chinese Medicine practitioners assuming that all channel types share the same general concepts. This is simply *not* the case, and the study of the channel system, known in Chinese Medicine as Jing Luo (经络), is a huge subject in its own right.

In fact, different methods of treatment would classically be used depending on which type of channel needed treating. For instance, the Cutaneous regions and the Sinew channels (being the most external aspects of the channel system) would be treated with external Herbal Medicine and bodywork therapies; the Luo connecting vessels would commonly be treated by the use of bloodletting; the Primary and Divergent channels would be treated through the use of Acupuncture and internal Herbal Medicine; and the Extraordinary vessels would be regulated through self-cultivation exercises such as internal alchemy (only much later in history was Acupuncture and Herbal Medicine used to regulate the Extraordinary vessels).

Classically, when a student would learn Chinese Medicine (which was mostly done through an apprenticeship-style situation), study of the Jing Luo would be done systematically, with each category of channels being taught individually as a completely separate entity. This method of learning would often start with the most exterior of the channel categories (a brief explanation of the channel categories can be found below), and the student would not move on to the next channel type until they had fully understood the one that they were currently learning. For instance, a student would begin by learning and understanding the Cutaneous regions, and only once the student fully understood the functions, behaviours and illnesses associated with the Cutaneous regions would they move on to the Sinew channels. Once they understood and essentially mastered the theories and also treatment of the Sinew channels, they would be then allowed to move on to the Luo (络) connecting channels, then the Primary channels, and so on. This progression in learning is also mirrored in the types of treatments used for each channel type (described above), as moving from bodywork to Acupuncture to Herbal Medicine and then eventually to internal alchemy, can also be seen as a progression in terms of difficulty and time spent needed to learn.

It should be noted that although understanding the Sinew channels is arguably the most important aspect of the channel system in regards to Tui Na (mainly due to the fact that it is the Sinew channels that we are directly affecting through Tui Na), that is not to say that the other channel types are not important. It is essential to understand the Primary channels, for instance, in order to use Tui Na to treat internal medical conditions, as the use of specific acupoints (found along the Primary channels) is necessary. Over the following pages, it will be the Sinew channels that are discussed in detail, as the Primary channels and acupoints with their associated functions and indications can be found readily in many other publications.

Categorisation of the channels and collaterals (Jing Luo, 经络)

The Sinew channels are classed as part of a larger collateral system within the channels and collaterals theory, along with the 12 Cutaneous regions and 16 Luo vessels. Although the whole of the Jing Luo system is classed as the 'exterior' within Chinese Medicine (with the 'interior' referring to the vital organs), the Cutaneous channels, Sinew channels and Luo (络) vessels are considered to be the exterior aspect of the Jing Luo system. With the nature of Tui Na (or any other bodywork therapy) being very physical and working on the exterior of the body, it is naturally the Cutaneous regions and the Sinew channels that we should be focusing on, with the Sinew channels having particular importance (with the Luo connecting channels being used more for bloodletting). As part of the more external aspect of the Jing Luo system, the Sinew channels do not directly connect with the internal vital organs, although because of their relationship with the Primary channels, they can have an indirect affect by altering the circulation and flow of Qi and Blood within the body.

As mentioned previously, they can also have an effect on the Shen (神), which again, will affect the functioning of the body as a whole. The following pages focus on the Sinew channels in greater depth, as I feel it is often overlooked yet fundamental to understand in order to take Tui Na from merely being a massage therapy to being a whole medical system.

Wei	Cutaneous regions (Pi Jing)	
	Sinew channels (Jing Jin)	
	Luo vessels (Luo Mai)	Exterior
Ying	- - - - - - - - - - - - -	Interior
	Primary channels (Hou Tian Jing)	
	Divergent channels (Jing Bie)	
Yuan	Extraordinary vessels (Qi Jing Ba Mai)	

Categorisation of the channels and collaterals (Jing Luo, 经络)

Introduction to the Sinew channels (Jing Jin, 经筋)

The Sinew channels are discussed in depth within the Chinese classics of medicine. They are introduced within the *Nei Jing Su Wen*, and have their own chapter within the *Ling Shu* (Chapter 13) that details their trajectories and also imbalances within the channels.

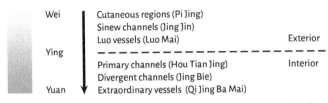

Chinese characters for Jing Jin (经筋)

The Chinese term for the Sinew channels is 'Jing Jin' (经筋). The term 'Jing' (经) means channel, or meridian, whereas 'Jin' (筋) is a collective term used for certain physical anatomical structures such as the sinews, tendons, muscles and fascia together. Other translations of Jing Jin include the Muscle channels, Tendino-Muscular channels, Tendon channels and Fascia channels, among others. Essentially they are the connective tissues of the body.

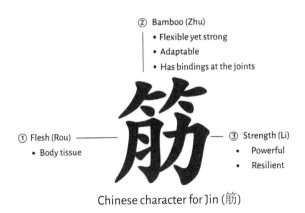

② Bamboo (Zhu)
 • Flexible yet strong
 • Adaptable
 • Has bindings at the joints

① Flesh (Rou)
 • Body tissue

③ Strength (Li)
 • Powerful
 • Resilient

Chinese character for Jin (筋)

It must be noted here that Jing Jin should actually be translated as channel Sinew rather than Sinew channel (which is how they are commonly known and how they will be referred to in this book). The importance of understanding that Jing Jin actually means channel Sinew rather than Sinew channel is mainly due to the fact that they should be seen as a connective series of tissues *belonging to* and *affecting* a channel, rather than simply a channel of connective tissue. This is a small yet vital linguistic differentiation to make. The Jing Jin are, in fact *not* channels, but the sinews associated with a channel. They should be seen as having a close relationship to the circulation of Qi and Blood through their associated primary channels, for example, the Lung channel, but also a physical structure in their own right with their own functions and dysfunctions. Understanding the Sinew channel theory as a completely separate entity of the channel system is a must for successful diagnostic and treatment outcomes.

Linguistics

Understanding that Jing Jin actually means channel Sinew rather than Sinew channel is a small yet vital distinction to make.

The Sinew channels do not follow direct and accurate pathways in the same way that the Primary channels do. As you will see later within the section on channel trajectories (see under 'The Sinew channels and diagnosis' later in this chapter), the Sinew channels are much broader and cover much wider areas. They overlap with one another, and interact together much more closely than the other channel categories, and cannot be located so precisely. What's more, unlike the varying directions of the Primary channels (depending if they are either a Yang channel or a Yin channel), *all Sinew channels originate at the extremities and flow upwards towards the head or the torso*. This is due to the fact that the Sinew channels are essentially governed by Wei Qi (a form of Yang Qi), and this is an important differentiation to make, especially when deciding to either tonify or reduce a channel.

Direction of flow

All Sinew channels originate at the extremities and flow towards the body.

The Sinew channels are what allow us to mobilise our tendons, muscles and ligaments, give the body activity (Yang), and keep us supported when resting (Yin). The Sinew channels are rarely taught or discussed within many Chinese Medicine courses (perhaps due to the focus on the Primary channels and Extraordinary channels within Acupuncture), although they are possibly the single most important channel category for Tui Na practitioners (and, of course, other bodyworkers such as Shiatsu practitioners and Western physical therapists). It is important to understand that their behaviour and functioning is entirely different to that of the Primary channels, and it is essential to not treat them in the same way that you would the channels that are used more commonly within Acupuncture.

An entirely different system

The Sinew channels act in an entirely different way to that of the Primary channels, and the theories of any channel category should not be treated as the same as each other, as is all too common in modern practice.

In modern times, to make things simpler, each of the Sinew channels has adopted the name of its associated organ channel, so, for example, the Arm Tai Yin Sinew channel has become the Lung Sinew channel and so on. Although there is absolutely no direct reference between the organs and the Sinew channels in classical literature, this has become the norm in modern texts, and I will also refer to each channel according to its associated organ channel. These names can be seen in the table below:

Sinew channel names	
Leg Tai Yang	Bladder Sinew channel
Arm Tai Yang	Small Intestine Sinew channel
Leg Shao Yang	Gall Bladder Sinew channel
Arm Shao Yang	San Jiao Sinew channel
Leg Yang Ming	Stomach Sinew channel
Arm Yang Ming	Large Intestine Sinew channel
Leg Tai Yin	Spleen Sinew channel
Arm Tai Yin	Lung Sinew channel
Leg Shao Yin	Kidney Sinew channel
Arm Shao Yin	Heart Sinew channel
Leg Jue Yin	Liver Sinew channel
Arm Jue Yin	Pericardium Sinew channel

Pairings and groupings of the Sinew channels

Learning about the Sinew channels makes us take a look at the body as a whole. The Sinew channels in this respect are effectively a collective term for the many muscles, tendons, sinews, fascia and all other connective tissues, and how they are related within the body. Once we get past the level of the skin (Cutaneous regions, see the categorisation above), we get to the Sinew channels. Along with the Cutaneous channels, the Sinew channels are an externalisation of the Primary channels, and act as a collateral to communicate with the Primary channels.

When discussing the Sinew channels, in addition to being referred to individually (for example, the Bladder Sinew channel or the Heart Sinew channel), they are also referred to as pairings or as groups of three. When discussing the Sinew channels as pairings, they may be referred to as the Tai Yang (Bladder and Small Intestine channels), the Shao Yang (Gall Bladder and San Jiao channels), the Yang Ming (Stomach and Large Intestine channels), the Tai Yin (Spleen and Lung channels), the Shao Yin (Kidney and Heart channels) or the Jue Yin (Liver and Pericardium channels). Each individual channel is then differentiated by being either an arm channel or leg channel, for instance, the Lung Sinew channel was classically called Arm Tai Yin Sinew channel, whereas the Spleen Sinew channel was called the Leg Tai Yin Sinew channel. These are named after the 'Six Divisions', essentially looking at each channel pairing as one larger channel that is split into an arm aspect and a leg aspect. It is important to note, however, that when thinking of these pairings according to the Six Divisions, they are not to be confused with the 'Six Conformations/Six Stages' in regards to diagnosis and disease progression, as this is an entirely different context, although the same terms are used.

When discussing the Sinew channels as groups of three, they may be referred to as the Leg Yang (Bladder, Gall Bladder and Stomach), the Arm Yang (Small Intestine, San Jiao and Large Intestine), the Leg Yin (Spleen, Kidney and Liver) and the Arm Yin (Lung, Heart and Pericardium).

Knowing these relationships is important, and the reason for this will become more apparent further into this discussion on the Sinew channels. A summary of each pairing and group of three can be found below:

Channel pairings	
Tai Yang	Bladder and Small Intestine channels
Shao Yang	Gall Bladder and San Jiao channels
Yang Ming	Stomach and Large Intestine channels
Tai Yin	Spleen and Lung channels
Shao Yin	Kidney and Heart channels
Jue Yin	Liver and Pericardium channels
Channel groupings	
Leg Yang	Bladder, Gall Bladder and Stomach channels
Arm Yang	Small Intestine, San Jiao and Large Intestine channels
Leg Yin	Spleen, Kidney and Liver channels
Arm Yin	Lung, Heart and Pericardium channels

Acupoints and the Sinew channels

The Sinew channels are not so point specific like the more interior channels such as Primary, Divergent and Extraordinary channels; however, all Sinew channels originate at the Jing Well points, which are located at certain points at the fingernails and toenails.

The Jing Well points are classed as the only standardised point on the Sinew channels, with all other points being what we call Ashi points (Ashi points are explained in more detail within Section 2). As mentioned previously when discussing tonification and reduction methods, because all channels begin at the Jing Well points, reinforcing a channel is generally going towards the body, whereas reducing is generally going away from the body.

Other points that are often discussed in regards to the Sinew channels are the 'Meeting Points' of the Sinew Channels, of which there are four. These are where certain combinations of the Sinew channels meet, and can be affected by the use of a single point on the body. For example, should a patient experience sciatica with discomfort affecting two or more of the Leg Yang channels (Bladder, Gall Bladder and Stomach), the point SI-18 (Quan Liao) may be used as this is where all three Leg Yang channels are said to meet. The same can apply to conditions affecting the three Leg Yin channels, the three Arm Yang channels and the three Arm Yin channels. The Meeting Points are often needled or stimulated in addition to the Jing Well point of the corresponding channel, and can be seen in the table below:

The four Meeting Points		
Meeting Point	Channel category	Sinew channels
GB-13	Three Leg Yang	Bladder, Gall Bladder, Stomach
R-3	Three Leg Yin	Spleen, Kidney, Liver
SI-18	Three Arm Yang	Small Intestine, San Jiao, Large Intestine
GB-22	Three Arm Yin	Lung, Heart, Pericardium

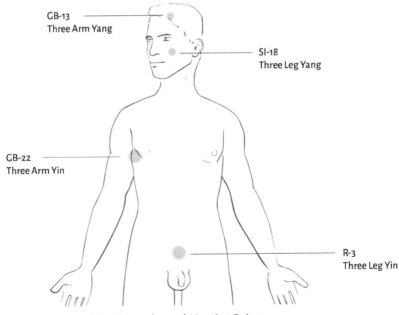

The Sinew channel Meeting Points

Functions of the Sinew channels as a whole

Taking into account all of the channel types, there are almost a hundred individual major channels within the body, and each one has its own unique function. However, each channel type also has a set of general functions that they share as a whole. As mentioned previously, these shared functions of each channel type are very different to another channel type. For instance, the general functions of the Primary channels are different to those of the Divergent channels, which are different to those of the Cutaneous regions and so on. The Sinew channels are no different, and each of the Sinew channels share a general function to help the self-regulation of the body. These functions can be found below (the functions of each individual Sinew channel can be found later in this section).

The Sinew channels protect the body's interior by circulating the Wei Qi (衛氣)

One of the main functions of the Sinew channels is to protect the body from external pathogens. From a Chinese Medicine perspective, external pathogens are commonly seen as the external climatic factors that are Wind, Heat, Cold, Dryness, Dampness and Summer Heat (sometimes referred to as Fire). In Chinese Medicine these are known as the Xie Qi (邪氣), meaning the Evil Qi (pathogens).

However, protecting the body from external pathogens also refers to external emotional factors, such as the influence of other people's emotions, which are also considered to be external pathogens. Other people's emotions and stress created by being in certain environments are classically also considered to be one of the three types of Wind invasion, the other two being the invasion of climatic Wind (discussed above), and the invasion of Heavenly Wind in the way of 'possession by spirits'. Wei Qi is what acts as our defence against these pathogens, with Wei Qi often being interpreted as 'defensive Qi' or 'protective Qi'. Due to the fact that the Sinew channels essentially act as conduits to the Wei Qi (see below for a further discussion on the Sinew channels and Wei Qi), the Sinew channels are seen to protect the body from these pathogenic factors.

In addition to protecting the body energetically from external pathogens, it is the Sinew channels that act as actual physical protection to the body. The muscles and tendons act as a type of natural body armour alongside our bone structure in order to protect our more vulnerable organs and structures, such as our vessels.

The Sinew channels govern movement

Just like the muscular system in Western medicine, the Sinew channels govern movement of the body and limbs from a Chinese Medicine perspective. This is perhaps the Sinew channels' most simple yet fundamental function. This not only refers to the physical action of activating and relaxing the soft tissues (such as muscles and tendons) in order to create contractions and therefore movement, but also refers again to the circulation of Wei Qi that gives the body animation and movement. When the Sinew channels are healthy and strong, the Wei Qi will circulate freely, allowing the body to move quickly and precisely, whilst also being able to move slowly, gently and for longer periods of time. When the Sinew channels are damaged, the Wei Qi cannot circulate properly, and there may be lack of movement or restricted movement that is jittery in motion. Movements may also be weakened and will lack endurance.

In addition to generating movement for the major muscle groups and the skeletal muscles, the Sinew channels also assist in the circulation of Wei Qi through to the smooth muscle within the body that helps in the autonomic functions of respiration (Lung), digestion (Spleen), circulation (Heart) and urination (Kidney). This shows how treatment of the Sinew channels, for instance, with Tui Na, can have an effect on regulating the Zang Fu and therefore the key autonomic functions of the body.

The Sinew channels keep stability and maintain posture

It is the Sinew channels that enable the body to keep stability and maintain its upright posture. By maintaining a balance of Yin and Yang (flexibility and strength, engagement and relaxation), the Sinew channels maintain the structure of the skeletal system in a way that allows the Qi and Blood to flow smoothly throughout the body. When the Sinew channels are working efficiently, our core will stabilise the spine and body, the legs will help to keep the body steady, and the arms will hold integrity to the shoulders, chest and neck. Should the Sinew channels be excess or deficient, however, opposing muscle groups will become out of balance, thus affecting the posture and therefore the circulation of Qi and Blood to various parts of the body.

General functions of the Sinew channels

- The Sinew channels protect the body's interior by circulating the Wei Qi (衛氣).

- The Sinew channels govern movement.

- The Sinew channels keep stability and maintain posture.

Relationship between the Sinew channels and the Primary channels

Although the Sinew channels and Primary channels are entirely different components of the body, they do indeed follow very similar pathways. In addition to the fact that the Sinew channels are not discussed at length within the modern study of Chinese Medicine, this is possibly the reason why many students and practitioners believe that the two types of channels share the same behaviours and functions. As mentioned above, the Sinew channels are essentially groups of muscles, tendons and connective tissues that are associated with and assist their corresponding Primary channel. The Primary channels also assist with the functioning of their associated Sinew channel. Qi and Blood of the Primary channels supply and nourish the Sinew channels, giving them functionality, nourishment and strength, whereas activation and movement of the Sinew channels encourages movement of Qi, Blood and Body Fluids throughout the Primary channels, and provides stability and structure to the channel pathways. The Sinew channels also act as both physical and energetic protection to the Primary channels due to the Sinew channels acting as conduits for the Wei Qi to circulate throughout the body.

When there is a deficiency within a Primary channel, such as insufficient Qi and Blood, there will likely be weakness and/or numbness in the Sinew channel. If there is stagnation of Qi and Blood in a Primary channel, this may give rise to pain, discomfort and/or numbness in a Sinew channel. Equally, if there is stagnation or injury to a Sinew channel, this will likely affect the flow of Qi and Blood within the Primary channels, whilst also leaving the Primary channels open to external pathogenic factors. Treatment of the Sinew channels will ultimately benefit the Primary channels, and vice versa.

Relationship between the Sinew channels and the Zang Fu (脏腑) organs

As we know from basic Chinese Medicine theory, everything that we do to the body on one level will have a similar effect at the other levels, be it the superficial level of the skin and sinews, the organ level, or even at the level of the mind and consciousness. The body is connected as one through the Jing Luo system. Therefore, by opening and relaxing the body at the superficial level, it will have the same effect at an organ level (and also the level of consciousness). Improving the Qi and Blood flow through the Sinew channels, although being energetically superficial, will essentially improve the Qi and Blood flow through to the associated organs.

Although each of the Sinew channels is named after a corresponding organ, it should be known that the Sinew channels have no *direct* connection to the associated internal Zang Fu (脏腑) organs, although they do, of course, have an indirect connection – communication between the two occurs mainly via the body's Primary channels in addition to the Huang (肓, membranes). For us to have a direct influence on the organs with Tui Na, we would need to use focused acupressure on specific acupoints that are located along the Primary channels. However, treatment of the Sinew channels can, of course, have an indirect effect on the Zang Fu through their influence on the circulation and flow of Qi and Blood, and therefore an interaction with the other channel types. For instance, by releasing tension in the Lung Sinew channel, this will have an influence on the flow of Qi and Blood of the Lung primary meridian and also open up the physical region of the Lungs, which can therefore have an effect on the vitality of the Lung Qi and the organ. What's more, working along the Lung Sinew channel will also help to release any tension within the Huang surrounding the Lungs, that will result in better Qi flow in and out of the Lungs.

Affecting the Zang Fu organs

For us to have a direct influence on the organs with Tui Na, we would need to use focused acupressure on specific acupoints that are located along the Primary channels. Working on the Sinew channels without stimulating specific points indirectly influences the internal organs by affecting the flow of Qi and Blood and releasing the Huang (肓, membranes).

The Sinew channels and Wei Qi (衛氣)

The *Ling Shu* describes three levels of Qi within the body – the Wei, Ying and Yuan. These levels generally refer to the exterior, interior and congenital layers of the body respectively. Other Chinese Medicine practitioners, such as herbalists, may refer to these levels as the Qi, Blood and Jing levels. In regards to the Sinew channels and the therapy of Tui Na, it is the Wei level that we are most interested in, which understandably is governed in particular by the Wei Qi.

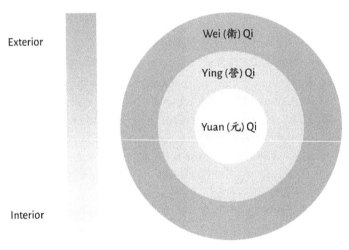

Three levels of Qi – Wei (衛), Ying (營) and Yuan (元)

Wei Qi is commonly interpreted as *defensive* Qi and is said to circulate outside of the vessels, within the spaces between the skin and the sinews that are known as the Cou Li (腠理). It is from our Kidney Yang that our Wei Qi originates, and it is therefore a form of Yang Qi. It is our Liver that ensures the Wei Qi flows smoothly through the Sinew channels, which essentially act as conduits. The key functions of Wei Qi can be found below:

Key functions of Wei Qi (衛氣)

- To promote warmth and movement within the channels.

- To control the exterior of our body to protect against external pathogens such as the six climatic factors (Wind, Cold, Heat, Damp, Dryness, and Summer Heat/Fire) and also externally projected emotions (classically also characterised as pathogenic Wind).

- To encourage healing of any damage caused by these factors.

It is thought that if our exterior and therefore our Wei Qi is strong, then our bodies won't surrender to disease. This does not only mean to be protected against external pathogenic factors such as the six climatic factors, but also to prevent any illness from internal disorders such as the emotions and internal diseases. This is because of the way that our Wei Qi can open the exterior and allow internal disorders to be released and vented through sweating and/or purging (physically and energetically). This is one reason why it is possible to experience an emotional release during or shortly after receiving a Tui Na treatment.

Conduits of Wei Qi (衛氣)

The Sinew channels are the conduits of the Wei Qi (衛氣, defensive Qi).

Wei Qi is involved in regulating many of the body's involuntary actions, such as the mechanism of breathing, sweating, heart rate and also peristalsis in regards to the digestive system, all through the stimulation of smooth muscle. It is also responsible for our instinctive actions such as our reflexes and involuntary reactions to the external environment. These are all aspects of the body that can be affected through treatment of the Sinew channels, and demonstrate how Tui Na is able to have an effect on the body's involuntary autonomic processes. Understanding these processes and the functions of Wei Qi also gives us a greater understanding and broader application of Tui Na when working on the Sinew channels, and in order to fully understand the extent to which Tui Na can help, understanding of at least the foundations of Chinese Medicine is fundamental.

The fact that the Sinew channels act as conduits of our Wei Qi means that the Sinew channels are most likely affected when there are disorders of the Wei Qi. For instance, when pathogenic Cold attempts to invade the body, such as when we catch the flu or the common cold, the Sinew channels will react and we will experience aching and uncomfortable movement due to the interaction between the Wei Qi and the pathogenic Qi. From an emotional point of view, if we experience a period of elevated stress, the Sinew channels again will become affected and we may experience tightness in the Sinew channels such as tight shoulders and neck (Wind causes contraction of the muscles and sinews).

The Lungs and Liver are the organs responsible for the regulation of the Wei Qi. The Lungs act through the breath and the skin, while the Liver acts through its control of the sinews and the free flow of Qi. Each of the Jing Well points (where each Sinew channel begins) is classed as either a Metal (Lung) or a Wood (Liver) point, indicating the important relationship between the Sinew channels and these organs, and therefore the regulation of Wei Qi. Both of these organs are affected by Wind (the Lungs are affected by external Wind, and the Liver is affected by internal Wind), and this explains why Wei Qi is also associated with Wind. This may indicate why it is said that treatment of the Sinew channels (and Cutaneous channels) helps protect against 'the 100 diseases', as Chapter 3 of the *Su Wen* states that 'Wind is the root of all perversity'.

A brief note on emotions

As discussed above, the actions of Wei Qi and the Sinew channels are automatic and unconscious. When our bodies react to situations or events in a certain way, and we don't know why, it is generally due to a 'memory' stored within our Sinew channels from an experience that we have previously had. It works in the same way that our muscles and tendons will react to pain, the anticipation of pain, or even a memory of pain, on a physical level. For instance, if a situation unconsciously reminds us of an experience that we had previously and did not like or felt that we needed protecting from, the Wei Qi will cause the Sinew channels to contract, causing us to feel somewhat uncomfortable and to react with an emotion at the Wei level. This would be a very mild and almost unnoticeable contraction of the channels, and give rise to an emotion that we feel yet do not quite understand why we feel it (also called a 'mood'). Certain prejudices work in a similar way, and are generally based on our past experiences or past observations of others. Saying that someone is 'closed-minded' because they are judgmental of a particular topic may, in fact, actually be true, that their Sinew channels are responding by restricting Qi and Blood flow, and therefore affecting the Shen, the mind.

In a similar respect, the body's emotional condition will reflect the condition of the Sinew channels, and our posture will likewise reflect our mood that we experience on the Wei level. For example, feeling sad could indicate hypertonicity of the Lung Sinew channels as the channel is preventing the emotion from being vented by obstructing the flow of Qi and Blood. This may manifest as a caved chest-like posture, with rounded and sunken shoulders. Working on the Sinew channels through bodywork can help to open up and give correct posture, and therefore evoke a release of these surface emotions, causing a change in mental state. It is for this reason that becoming familiar with the core emotions (Anger, Joy, Pensiveness, Sadness/Grief and Fear/Fright) and their associated elemental energetics or channels is important.

The sequence of Qi flow within the Sinew channels

The circulation of Wei Qi does not match the flow of Qi that is typically discussed with the Primary channels (also discussed as the Channel Clock theory), but follows the Sinew channel sequence over a 24-hour period. Again, unlike the circulation of Qi through the Primary channels, the circulation through the Sinew channels does not begin in the Lungs at around 3am regardless, but is activated at the point BL-1 when we open our eyes after sleeping. This is why it important to find out when the patient generally wakes up day to day to determine which channels are more engaged at which times. The Wei Qi will flow through the Yang channels during the day, and the Yin channels during the night over a 24-hour period.

The sequence of the Sinew channels begins with the Leg Yang channels (moving in order through the Bladder Tai Yang, Gall Bladder Shao Yang and then the Stomach Yang Ming), then moves in order through the Arm Yang Channels (Small Intestine Tai Yang, San Jiao Shao Yang, then the Large Intestine Yang Ming). Once it has circulated through the Yang channels, it circulates in order through the Spleen and Lung Tai Yin channels, Kidney and Heart Shao Yin channels, and finishes in the Liver and Pericardium Jue Yin channels. A summary of this sequence can be seen below:

Sequence of the flow of Wei Qi (衛氣)

Yang channels: Bladder – Gall Bladder – Stomach – Small Intestine – San Jiao – Large Intestine

Yin channels: Spleen – Lung – Kidney – Heart – Liver – Pericardium

---

The importance of understanding this sequence is that, due to the circulation of Wei Qi, this is also the sequence that ailments can spread from one channel to another (for example, through structural compensation or spreading of pathogens). It is also the sequence in which the body should be treated in order to resolve these issues. For instance, if someone has an injury or ailment affecting the Stomach Sinew channel, if left untreated this may begin to affect the surrounding channels within the sequence, and continue to spread deeper throughout the sequence over time (initially spreading to the Small Intestine channel and so on). What's more, treatment of the Stomach Sinew channel would classically involve treatment of the Stomach channel, followed by the Gall Bladder, and then the Bladder channel, working backwards through the sequence, until the ailment has been resolved.

Order of treatment

When multiple channels are affected, it is important that we treat the most interior of the channels first (determined from the order stated above).

An arguably less important sequence of the Sinew channels is that of the seasons. As mentioned above, the circulation of Wei Qi happens every 24 hours, and begins when we open our eyes after sleeping, travelling through the Yang channels during the day and the Yin channels during the night. However, in addition to the sequence of Wei Qi, there is another sequence that occurs over a 12-month period in accordance with the seasons, and refers to specific channels being more prone to afflictions at certain times of the year. This is discussed in Chapter 13 of the *Ling Shu*. It should be noted, however, that although this sequence explains when ailments are most likely to happen, ailments of any channel can occur at any time of year. The sequence is said to begin with the Bladder Tai Yang channel suffering from conditions known as Zhong Chun Bi (Middle Spring Painful Blockage Syndrome). Chapter 13 of the *Ling Shu* then discusses the following sequence, all referring to Bi (痹, painful blockage) syndromes during specific times of the year.

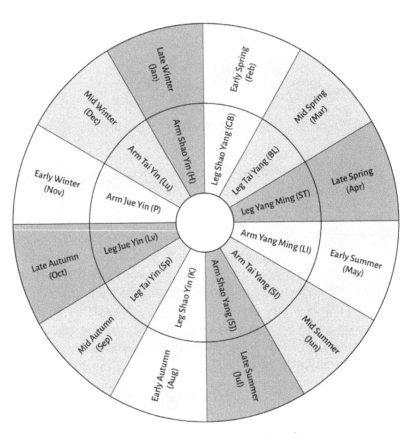

Sequence of the Sinew channels throughout the seasons

The Sinew channels and external pathogenic factors

Due to the fact that Sinew channels act as the first line of defence to the body against external pathogenic factors, they are easily affected by external pathogens and can suffer from disorders caused by them. Each pathogenic factor causes the Sinew channels to 'react' in a different way, and therefore causes different symptoms and signs depending on which pathogen(s) is causing the disruption. Although it is generally considered that there are six external pathogens (Wind, Cold, Damp, Heat, Summer Heat/Fire, Dryness), only three of them tend to affect the Sinew channels in a way that causes disorder to them – these are Wind, Cold and Damp, or various combinations of the three. It should be noted that these pathogens may only enter the Sinew channels and cause injury if the Wei Qi is deficient and weaker than the pathogenic Qi. It should also be noted here that Heat also affects the Sinew channels – not as a pathogen, but as a result of the arrival of Wei Qi due to trauma in need of repair.

Pathogenic Qi

The external pathogens may only enter the Sinew channels and cause injury if the Wei Qi is deficient and weaker than the pathogenic Qi.

Wind (风, Feng)

The Wind pathogen is considered Yang, due to its moving and sudden onset nature. As Wind enters the Sinew channels, it causes them to contract, in the same way that we may get a stiff neck if we sit next to a draught. Due to the fact that Wind causes contraction of the Sinew channels, it can also cause them to tremor or quiver. If the Wind pathogen is causing pain in the Sinew channels, the pain usually wanders around unpredictably, as is the behaviour of Wind in nature.

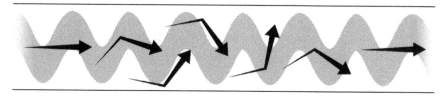

Unpredictable and rapid nature of pathogenic Wind

Cold (寒, Han)

The Cold pathogen is considered Yin in nature, due to its contracting, stagnating and slow onset nature. Like Wind, Cold also causes the tendons to contract. However, the tendons do not contract so suddenly or quickly as they would with Wind. What's more, rather than a quiver or a tremor (as experienced with the Wind pathogen), the contraction as a result of Cold will cause slow, tense and stiff movements. If there is pain, this may be categorised as a sharp, stabbing pain of fixed location, much like frostbite, and the pain will be alleviated by warmth. The patient may also feel an aversion to Cold, and the tissues local to the injury site may be pale, or pale with a blue tinge.

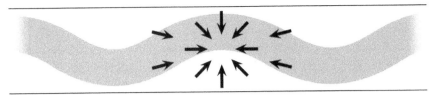

Stagnating and contracting nature of pathogenic Cold

Damp (湿, Shi)

The Damp pathogen is also considered Yin in nature due to its heavy, stagnating and substantial nature. When Damp builds up and affects the Sinew channels, the patient will experience heaviness and lethargy in the movements activated by the affected channels. If there is pain, this may be categorised as a dull ache. There may also be swelling in the area, and also numbness locally or distally, due to the Damp obstructing the flow of Qi and Blood.

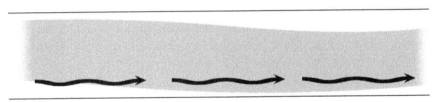

Heavy, sluggish and substantial nature of pathogenic Damp

Damp can also mix with Heat, which is created as a side effect of the arrival of Wei Qi to an injury site, to create Damp Heat within the Sinew channels. This would manifest with the signs stated above with Damp, and in addition with the feeling of warmth, radiating pain and/or redness. The patient may feel relief by the application of Cold and also have an aversion to warmth.

Pathogen	Symptoms and signs affecting the Sinew channels
Wind	Sudden onset; sudden contraction of tendons that may or may not cause tremor; wandering pain
Cold	Gradual onset; contraction of sinews and tendons causing tension and stiffness; sharp, stabbing pain of fixed location; pale/bluish tinge to the surrounding tissues, feeling of cold; aversion to warmth; relief by the application of warmth
Damp	Heaviness and lethargy; sluggish movement; dull ache; swelling; numbness

The Sinew channels and diagnosis

Diagnosis of the Sinew channels is not done through tongue or pulse, but is generally achieved through palpation, range of movement and channel strength/engagement. Observation and understanding of how the body moves in both a healthy and unhealthy manner is important. Below is a brief summary of diagnosis using the Sinew channels, although more detailed information can be found in Section 2.

Palpation

Palpating along areas of the body is essential in order to correctly diagnose areas of dysfunction. Generally speaking, the location of pain as perceived by the patient is not an indicator of the root of the problem. It is important to get hands on, along with understanding the trajectories of the channels, and palpate along a channel and its related channels. We need to consider, is the channel tight (excess)? Is the channel weak (deficient)? Are there any Ashi points? (See Section 2 for an explanation on Ashi points.) Is it more or less painful on palpation? There are many questions that you can ask yourself during palpation that will build a comprehensive diagnosis based on Chinese Medicine principles. More will be discussed about palpation and diagnosis in Section 2.

Range of movement

As obvious as it may seem, it is important to first understand a normal, healthy anatomical range of movement for any given part of the body. It is no good trying to help someone who can't move their arm in a certain way when it shouldn't even do it in the first place! (You would be surprised how many patients complain of lack of movement, when, in fact, they shouldn't be able to move in that way anyway.) It is also important to examine and assess the range of movement for each patient: is there too little movement (hypomobility)? Or is there too much movement (hypermobility)? This can tell us the health of the Sinew channels, and the quality of the Qi and Blood. More will be discussed about the movements of each channel later in this section, whilst range of movement and diagnosis of each Sinew channel, along with special examinations, can be found in Section 2 of this book.

Channel strength/engagement

It is also important to test the engagement of affected channels (or if there is time, all channels), and the strength of each channel in various planes of movement. Ultimately, it is best to recreate everyday movements, and to recreate the movements that are causing discomfort and explore any other movements that the patient may not have realised are problematic. By performing strength/engagement testing, we are able to find out channel imbalances and weaknesses of specific or numerous channels. We can then use this in order to direct our treatment principles.

For example, when a Yin channel is overactive (excess) or hypertonic, it may tell us that the associated Yang channel will be inactive (deficient), or vice versa.

Signs and symptoms of the Sinew channels

Due to the fact that the Sinew channels are classed as the exterior of the body, signs and symptoms of the Sinew channels mainly include external disorders such as rheumatism, arthritis, pain and discomfort, restricted mobility and joint issues. Additionally, because the Sinew channels are situated on the exterior of the body, they are greatly influenced by external factors. This would include both climatic factors (such as people experiencing changes in symptoms with the weather and being able to 'feel' imminent weather changes), as well as external emotional factors such as tensions in the channels being aggravated by external stress or perceived threat. As mentioned whilst discussing the general functions of the Sinew channels, one of the main functions of the Sinew channels is to protect the body against external pathogens, which is why many disorders of the Sinew channels involve invasion of these pathogenic factors. Signs and symptoms of each specific channel can be found later in this section, when discussing each channel individually.

Channel trajectories

The channel trajectories show the pathways and distribution of the Sinew channels, and how they interact with the various joints and junctions of the body. It is important to understand the pathways of each channel in order to show how a dysfunction of one part of the body can affect, or be affected by, another part of the body. It is also important to understand the trajectories in order to treat the body as a whole, rather than focusing on a small area of the body. For example, if a patient presents with carpal tunnel syndrome, it is far too common in modern practice that treatment is focused on the wrist and hand. The cause of the condition is actually likely to have started further up the arm and possibly even on to the torso, and treatment of the whole channel is necessary for a full recovery. Similarly, if the cause of the issue is indeed located around the wrist and hand, it is still essential to work on the associated channel up the arm and on to the torso, in order to increase the effectiveness of the treatment by opening the channels to allow space for healing and to promote a better flow of Qi and Blood to the areas.

Woven nature of the Sinew channels

It is important to note that, despite the appearance of many channel charts (including the ones within this book), the Sinew channels are not simply flat, two-dimensional lines that provide a 'layer' of the body. They are, in fact, three-dimensional, and are woven throughout the body to the deepest layers. The Yang Sinew channels tend to be more superficial, whereas the Yin channels travel deep to the core of the body for stabilisation, and connect to the Huang (肓, membranes) that surround the tissues and protect the organs.

It is actually very difficult to truly know which muscles and tendons are affected by specific channels, as it is not as simple as listing which muscles and tendons are located along a specific trajectory. It is also about which muscles and tendons are activated by the engagement of each specific Sinew channel. This can only be experienced through muscle testing and movement, and also through stretching and feeling the channels for yourself! However, later in this section I have listed a number of muscles and tendons that are situated along the specific pathways of a channel and that are also known to be activated by a specific channel. These can be found within the discussions of each individual channel, and should prove useful for those who are already trained in Western anatomy or Western bodywork therapies, and also for situations where a patient will come into the clinic complaining of an injury to a specific muscle or tendon using Western anatomical terminology.

The Sinew channel theory demonstrates the importance of both local and distal treatment. When treating a neck injury, for instance, it is all too simple to use Tui Na on the neck and perhaps the shoulder and upper back (all being local areas to the injury site). Using channel theory, we can see that it is necessary to also work down the arm to the hands, and also down the body as far as the feet (depending on what we find in diagnosis and which channel(s) are affected). This is because tension or issues anywhere along these channels, no matter how distal, is likely to affect the neck. Another example would be carpal tunnel syndrome. In my clinic, I hear too often of a patient going to see other healthcare professionals with carpal tunnel syndrome and the treatment being solely focused on the hand and wrist – the forearm, if they are lucky. There may be some temporary relief with this type of treatment, but ultimately the problem is unlikely to be confined to this small area, even if this is the only area that the patient feels discomfort. Truly successful treatment may require work to open up the channels from the neck, through the shoulder and elbow, and eventually into the wrist and hand. The carpal tunnel does not become constricted by itself for no reason – it is often due to tension further up the channel and can, indeed, be up as far as the neck and head. It is through understanding the Sinew channel theory that we know this.

Over the following pages you will find the general channel trajectories of each of the 12 Sinew channels.

Leg Tai Yang (Bladder) Sinew channel

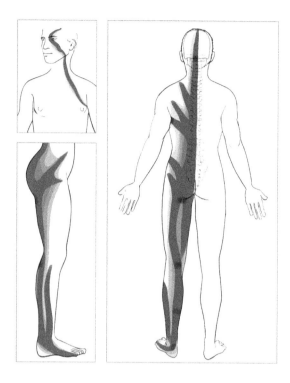

According to Chapter 13 of the *Ling Shu*, the sinews of the Bladder channel originate at the little toe, ascend and bind to the lateral malleolus, and continue up towards the knee. A branch separates at the binding at the lateral malleolus, extends to the heel, and rises upwards to bind at the lateral side of the popliteal fossa. Yet another branch separates at the binding of the lateral malleolus, ascends along the lateral side of the gastrocnemius, to bind at the medial side of the popliteal fossa. From here, it joins the previous branch in the gluteal region, and both branches ascend along the side of the spine towards the nape of the neck. Here, a branch enters the root of the tongue. Another branch emerges from the nape of the neck and binds at the occipital bone, ascends to the vertex of the head, and descends anteriorly to the cheek and binds to the bridge of the nose. Another branch circles around the eye.

A branch starts from the lateral side of the body, posterior to the armpit, and binds at the point Jian Yu (LI-15). Another branch enters the region below the armpit, and emerges by the supraclavicular fossa and binds at Wan Gu (GB-12). Another branch emerges from the supraclavicular fossa, obliquely ascends, and emerges at the side of the nose.

Western anatomy associated with the Bladder Sinew channel

The major muscles and tendons, in regards to Western anatomy, that are associated with the trajectory and activation of the Bladder Sinew channel are as follows (listed in alphabetical order):

- Abductor digiti minimi
- Biceps femoris
- Buccinator
- Compressor nares
- Corrugator supercilii
- Dilator nares
- Dorsal interosseous
- Erector spinae
- Extensor digitorum brevis
- Flexor digitorum longus
- Flexor halucis longus
- Frontalis
- Gastrocnemius
- Glutes
- Iliocostalis lumborum, thoracis
- Iliotibial tract
- Infraspinatus
- Lateral soleus
- Latissimus dorsi
- Levator anguli oris
- Levator costarum
- Levator labii superioris
- Levator scapulae
- Longissimus thoracis
- Masseter
- Medial pterygoid
- Occipitals
- Omohyoid
- Orbicularis oculi
- Pectoralis major and minor
- Peroneus brevis, longus, tertius
- Piriformis
- Plantaris
- Platysma
- Popliteus
- Posterior deltoid
- Procerus
- Risorius
- Scalene
- Semimembrinosus
- Semispinalis captis
- Semitendinosus
- Serratus
- Serratus posterior interior, superior
- Soleus
- Spinalis thoracis
- Splenius captis, cervicus
- Sternocleidomastoid
- Supraspinatus
- Teres major
- Tibialis posterior
- Trapezius
- Zygomaticus

Note: The actual muscles and tendons associated with the Bladder Sinew channel may indeed be more extensive than the list above. Due to the complex nature of functional movement, it is difficult to determine exactly which individual muscles and tendons are involved with each specific Sinew channel. The above list of muscles and tendons is based on clinical experience and observation in addition to anatomical understanding and modern research on the musculoskeletal system, and includes only major components of the musculoskeletal system. It is also important to note that some muscles and tendons will indeed be associated with multiple Sinew channels.

Mechanisms and movements of the Bladder Sinew channel

The Bladder Sinew channel is the leg aspect of the Tai Yang channel. The Tai Yang channels are located on the posterior aspect of the body, and are mainly related to our ability to stand up straight and give the movement of extension. It is the Bladder Sinew channel that gives us a strong posture and the ability to stand tall, with the head held high, which is also why the Bladder channel is linked closely to our self-esteem and self-confidence. The Bladder Sinew channel works closely with the Stomach Sinew channel in maintaining stability in the posture, and it is essential that both are balanced for powerful and stable movements.

Bladder Sinew channel

The movement of the Bladder Sinew channel can be clearly seen when we stand up from a seated position. It activates as the back straightens and the head lifts and looks forward. The action of lifting objects from the floor into a standing position, jumping forwards and upwards, and (to a certain extent) pulling objects inwards is also related to the Bladder Sinew channel.

Symptoms and signs of the Bladder Sinew channel

If the Bladder Sinew channel is weak, then the posture will collapse and the patient will look hunched over. There may be difficulty standing up straight, and extension of the back may be slow and uncomfortable or painful. There may also be difficulty in looking upwards.

If there is excessive tension in the Bladder Sinew channel, there may either be a forward or backward tilt in the pelvis (depending on which part of the channel is tight). There may also be difficulty and discomfort in looking down, and difficulty in bending forward or placing the legs out in front.

Classically, symptoms and signs of the Bladder Sinew channel are said to be worse during the middle of Spring (February), and include pain that occurs on extension, stiffness or discomfort that occurs when standing upright from a seated position, or an inability to stand tall. According to Chapter 13 of the *Ling Shu*, there may be paralysis of the little toe, swelling and discomfort in the heel, muscle pain and/or spasms experienced in the popliteal fossa, painful extension of the spine, stiffness in the occipital region, difficulty in raising the shoulder and muscle spasms of the axilla extending to the supraclavicular fossa.

Leg Shao Yang (Gall Bladder) Sinew channel

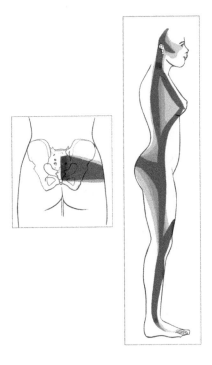

According to Chapter 13 of the *Ling Shu*, the sinews of the Gall Bladder channel begin at the fourth toe and ascend to bind at the lateral malleolus. They then ascend along the lateral side of the tibia, and bind at the lateral side of the knee. A branch starts from the lateral side of the fibula and ascends towards the thigh. Its anterior branch binds at Fu Tu (ST-32), and its posterior branch binds at the sacrum. A branch ascends through the ribs, runs along the anterior side of the armpit, connects to the chest and breast, and binds at the supraclavicular fossa. Another branch extends from the armpit and ascends through the supraclavicular fossa, emerges in front of the Bladder Sinew channel, travels upwards behind the ear and towards the temple. From here, it ascends to the angle of the forehead and meets at the vertex. It then descends to the mandible and binds at the side of the nose. Another branch binds at the outer canthus of the eye as the eye's external defence.

Western anatomy associated with the Gall Bladder Sinew channel

The major muscles and tendons, in regards to Western anatomy, that are associated with the trajectory and activation of the Gall Bladder Sinew channel are as follows (listed in alphabetical order):

- Biceps femoris
- Extensor digitorum brevis
- Frontalis
- Gluteus minimus
- Iliotibial band
- Obliques
- Pernoeus tirtius
- Piriformis
- Scalenus anterior
- Superior serratus anterior
- Temporalis
- Tensor fascia latae
- Transerse abdominis

Note: The actual muscles and tendons associated with the Gall Bladder Sinew channel may indeed be more extensive than the list above. Due to the complex nature of functional movement, it is difficult to determine exactly which individual muscles and tendons are involved with each specific Sinew channel. The above list of muscles and tendons is based on clinical experience and observation in addition to anatomical understanding and modern research on the musculoskeletal system, and includes only major components of the musculoskeletal system. It is also important to note that some muscles and tendons will indeed be associated with multiple Sinew channels.

Mechanisms and movements of the Gall Bladder Sinew channel

The Gall Bladder Sinew channel is the leg aspect of the Shao Yang channel. The Shao Yang channels are located mainly along the lateral aspects of the body, and govern the movement of rotation. The Shao Yang channels are associated with being the 'pivot' (Shao Yang Wei Shu, 少阳为枢), and do so between the exterior and the interior, or the Yang and the Yin aspects of the body. Energetically, the Gall Bladder channel is said to help us with our decision-making and freedom of thought, and having the courage to externalise those decisions and giving us direction. This can be seen physically by the Sinew channels governing rotation and enabling the body to change direction at will. It is also the Gall Bladder Sinew channel that helps to keep the body in alignment in regards to rotation of the hips and the legs, and balancing the Yin and Yang relationship of the body.

Gall Bladder Sinew channel

The movement of the Gall Bladder Sinew channels can be clearly seen when we rotate our body at the waist, and also when turning our legs and feet inwards or outwards from the hip. The Gall Bladder Sinew channel also activates lateral abduction of the legs.

Symptoms and signs of the Gall Bladder Sinew channel

If the Gall Bladder Sinew channel becomes tight or excessive, then the channel will pull along the lateral aspect of the glutes and upper leg, causing the foot to turn outwards. There will be pain or discomfort in the lower back and the hip, as the leg will not be aligned properly. This can be clearly seen when a patient is lying down in a supine position, and the feet are pointed in a direction of around 30 to 45 degrees laterally. Tightness in the Gall Bladder Sinew channel may also give rise to difficulty and discomfort in twisting the upper body at the waist, and also in side bending at the waist.

When the Gall Bladder Sinew channel is weak, the legs and feet may turn inwards, and the patient will also have very little power in the hips when turning. This can lead on to lower back pain and misalignment of the tissues that help with core stability.

Classically, symptoms and signs of the Gall Bladder Sinew channel are said to be worse during the early Spring (January), and include pain and stiffness that occurs on rotation of the legs and main trunk of the body. According to Chapter 13 of the *Ling Shu*, diseases of the Gall Bladder Sinew channel may include pain and/or spasm of the fourth toe that radiates from the lateral aspect of the knee, inability of the stretching and flexion of the knee, pain and/or spasm of the popliteal fossa that includes the hip and/or the sacral region, referred pain and discomfort in the hypochondrium and tissues of the chest, and inability to open the eyes due to tension in the sinews passing over the head.

Leg Yang Ming (Stomach) Sinew channel

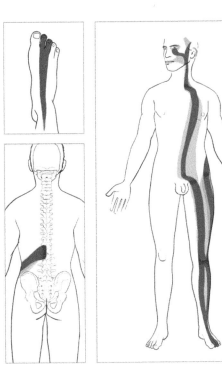

According to Chapter 13 of the *Ling Shu*, the sinews of the Stomach channel begin at the second, middle and fourth toes, bind at the dorsum of the foot, obliquely ascend along the lateral side of the fibula, and bind at the lateral side of the knee. From there, they ascend directly upwards to bind at the hip. They then extend to the lower ribs to connect with the spine. A straight branch travels along the tibia and binds at the knee. This branch binds at the fibula and joins with the Sinew channel of the Gall Bladder.

A straight branch ascends to the thigh, binds at the hip, and converges over the external genitalia. It then runs upwards to spread over the abdomen and binds at the supraclavicular fossa. From here it ascends to the neck and mouth, meets at the side of the nose and descends to bind at the nose. Here it joins the Bladder Sinew channel. The Bladder Sinew channel forms the upper muscular net around the eye, whereas the Stomach Sinew channel forms the lower muscular net around the eye. A branch stems from the cheek and binds in front of the ear.

Western anatomy associated with the Stomach Sinew channel

The major muscles and tendons, in regards to Western anatomy, that are associated with the trajectory and activation of the Stomach Sinew Channel are as follows (listed in alphabetical order):

- Adductors
- Buccinator
- Dorsal interossei
- Extensor digitorum brevis, longus
- Extensor hallucis brevis, longus
- Iliacus
- Iliopsoas
- Infrahyoids
- Internal and external obliques
- Latissimus dorsi
- Masseter
- Orbicularis oculi, oris
- Pectoralis major
- Peroneus brevis, longus, tertius
- Platysma
- Psoas
- Pterygoids
- Pyramidalis
- Rectus abdominis
- Sartorius
- Scalenes
- Soleus
- Sternocleidomastoid
- Subclavicus
- Suprahyoids
- Temporalis
- Tensor fascia latae
- Tibialis anterior
- Transverse abdominis
- Zygomaticus

Note: The actual muscles and tendons associated with the Stomach Sinew channel may indeed be more extensive than the list above. Due to the complex nature of functional movement, it is difficult to determine exactly which individual muscles and tendons are involved with each specific Sinew channel. The above list of muscles and tendons is based on clinical experience and observation in addition to anatomical understanding and modern research on the musculoskeletal system, and includes only major components of the musculoskeletal system. It is also important to note that some muscles and tendons will indeed be associated with multiple Sinew channels.

Mechanisms and movements and function of the Stomach Sinew channel

The Stomach Sinew channel is the leg aspect of the Yang Ming channel. The Yang Ming channels are located on the anterior aspect of the body, and are mainly related to our ability to brace ourselves and to bear weight, in addition to reaching out in front of us or pushing away.

The Stomach channel also maintains a Yin/Yang (front/back) relationship with the Bladder Sinew channels in assisting the Bladder Sinew channel to keep our posture strong and upright, especially when standing still. They essentially work together in the same way that we understand our core works with our back to maintain a stable posture.

Stomach Sinew channel

The movement of the Stomach Sinew channel can be clearly seen when a baby is learning to crawl, with the legs used to push away and propel the body forwards whilst bracing the core. (It is said within Chinese Medicine, that a child will develop their ability to stand strong through the act of crawling.)

Symptoms and signs of the Stomach Sinew channel

Symptoms and signs of the Stomach Sinew channel are classically said to be worse during the late Spring (March), and include the inability to stand still without discomfort or pain. The patient will be forced to collapse at the waist when standing still, and will not be able to hold any weight out in front of them (the patient should, however, feel okay to stand up straight when walking forward due to the Tai Yang channels taking over; this is a key diagnostic sign of Stomach Sinew channel dysfunction). Due to the trajectory passing through the jaw and on to the cheekbones, misalignment of the jaw may occur when there is Cold or tension within the upper aspects of the Sinew channel. According to Chapter 13 of the *Ling Shu*, there may be muscle spasms experienced in the third toe and/or the rectus femoris, foot and ankle stiffness with difficulty in jumping actions, swelling in the upper thigh, scrotal swelling and inguinal hernia, spasms of the abdomen extending to the supraclavicular fossa and cheek, and sudden misalignment of the upper and lower jaws.

Arm Tai Yang (Small Intestine) Sinew channel

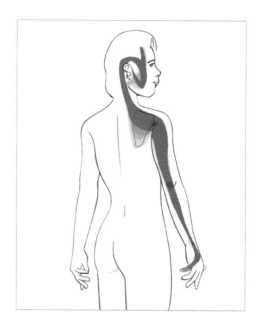

According to Chapter 13 of the *Ling Shu*, the sinews of the Small Intestine channel start at the tip of the little finger and bind at the wrist. They then ascend along the medial side of the forearm and bind at the medial epicondyle of the humerus. When knocked, a sensation of numbness is felt radiating to the little finger. From here, the channel ascends and binds below the axilla. Its branch runs behind the axilla and curves around the scapula, ascends along the neck to emerge in front of the Bladder Sinew channel, and binds at the mastoid process behind the ear. Another branch enters the ear. The straight branch emerges from the ear, binds at the mandible and connects with the outer canthus.

Western anatomy associated with the Small Intestine Sinew channel

The major muscles and tendons, in regards to Western anatomy, that are associated with the trajectory and activation of the Small Intestine Sinew channel are as follows (listed in alphabetical order):

- Abductor digiti minimi
- Anconeus
- Auriculares
- Extensor carpi ulnaris
- Flexor carpi ulnaris
- Infraspinatus
- Lateral and medial pterygoids
- Levator scapulae
- Masseter
- Orbicularis oculi
- Posterior deltoid
- Rhomboids (major and minor)

- Serratus
- Subscapularis
- Supraspinatus
- Temporalis
- Temporoparitalis

- Teres major
- Teres minor
- Trapezius
- Triceps brachii
- Zygomaticus

Note: The actual muscles and tendons associated with the Small Intestine Sinew channel may indeed be more extensive than the list above. Due to the complex nature of functional movement, it is difficult to determine exactly which individual muscles and tendons are involved with each specific Sinew channel. The above list of muscles and tendons is based on clinical experience and observation in addition to anatomical understanding and modern research on the musculoskeletal system, and includes only major components of the musculoskeletal system. It is also important to note that some muscles and tendons will indeed be associated with multiple Sinew channels.

Mechanisms and movements of the Small Intestine Sinew channel

The Small Intestine Sinew channel is the arm aspect of the Tai Yang channel. The Tai Yang channels are located on the posterior aspect of the body, and essentially give us the ability to stabilise whilst giving the movement of extension.

Small Intestine Sinew channel

Key movements of the Small Intestine Sinew channel can be clearly seen when lifting the arm up and extending it outwards in front (with extension travelling through the little finger), as if reaching out for something. Another common action of the Small Intestine Sinew channel is to hold the arms up and forwards in order to hold on to a steering wheel, or in order to type at a computer. It is also the Small Intestine Sinew channel that gives us correct engagement of the scapula and stabilises the entire shoulder joint through the rotator cuff.

Symptoms and signs of the Small Intestine Sinew channel

When the Small Intestine Sinew channels are injured, the patient will feel discomfort in and around the scapula area that will be made worse when lifting the arms upwards in front of them. Actions such as driving and using a computer will make symptoms worse, and pain may radiate upwards into the neck. Patients may also have limited movement in the shoulder joint, and have instability of the shoulder joint when lifting objects above the head.

Symptoms and signs of the Small Intestine Sinew channel are classically said to be worse during the mid-Summer (June). According to Chapter 13 of the *Ling Shu*, diseases of the Small Intestine Sinew channel may include stiffness of the little finger, pain in the posterior side of the humerus at the elbow that may radiate up the medial arm towards the posterior axillary fold, pain below the armpit, referred pain around the scapula and neck, pain and tinnitus in the ear, referred pain towards the mandible, blurred vision, inability of the eyes to focus quickly, and spasm of the neck muscles along the channel trajectory.

Arm Shao Yang (San Jiao) Sinew channel

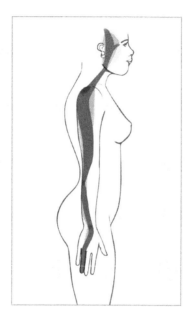

According to Chapter 13 of the *Ling Shu*, the sinews of the San Jiao channel start at the tip of the fourth finger and bind at the dorsum of the hand. They then ascend along the forearm and bind at the olecranon of the elbow. From here, they run upwards along the lateral side of the upper arm, ascend to the shoulder and on to the neck, and finally join with the Small Intestine Sinew channel. Its branch emerges from the angle of the mandible and connects with the root of the tongue. Another branch ascends to Jia Che (ST-6), runs in the front of the ear and connects with the outer canthus. It then runs upward to the mandible and binds at the corner of the forehead.

Western anatomy associated with the San Jiao Sinew channel

The major muscles and tendons, in regards to Western anatomy, that are associated with the trajectory and activation of the San Jiao Sinew Channel are as follows (listed in alphabetical order):

- Biceps brachii
- Buccinator
- Dorsal interosseous
- Extensor carpi ulnaris

- Extensor digiti minimi
- Extensor digitorum profundus
- Extensor digitorum superficialis
- Extensor indicis
- Lateral deltoid
- Masseter
- Medial pterygoid
- Orbucularis oculi
- Platysma
- Sternocleidomastoid
- Temporalis
- Trapezius
- Triceps brachii

Note: The actual muscles and tendons associated with the San Jiao Sinew channel may indeed be more extensive than the list above. Due to the complex nature of functional movement, it is difficult to determine exactly which individual muscles and tendons are involved with each specific Sinew channel. The above list of muscles and tendons is based on clinical experience and observation in addition to anatomical understanding and modern research on the musculoskeletal system, and includes only major components of the musculoskeletal system. It is also important to note that some muscles and tendons will indeed be associated with multiple Sinew channels.

Mechanisms and movements of the San Jiao Sinew channel

The San Jiao Sinew channel is the arm aspect of the Shao Yang channel. The Shao Yang channels are located at the sides of the body, and are related essentially to our body's ability to rotate on a central axis. The Shao Yang is considered as the 'pivot' of the Yang channels, as stated in Chapter 6 of the *Su Wen* (Shao Yang Wei Shu, 少阳为枢). This includes free rotation of the torso, rotation of the limbs, and rotation and side bending of the neck/head.

San Jiao Sinew channel

The movement of the San Jiao Sinew channel can be clearly seen in rotation of the arms on a central axis (in a pronating/supinating manner such as using a screwdriver or turning a door handle), lateral abduction of the arm, and turning or tilting the head to one side. It also assists in the movement of the opening and closing of the jaw and movement of the tempo-mandibular joint due to the channel trajectory passing over the lower jaw and in front of the ears.

Symptoms and signs of the San Jiao Sinew channel

When the San Jiao Sinew channels are injured, rotation of the upper aspects of the body such as the head, neck and upper limbs will be affected. This will cause the patient to be unable to rotate or laterally tilt the head without discomfort. Injury to the San Jiao Sinew channel will also cause the patient discomfort in performing arm rotation movements such as using a screwdriver or opening jars and turning door handles. In these actions, pain will usually manifest at the Sinew channel binding sites, such as the elbow and/or shoulder. Tightness in the San Jiao Sinew channel may also manifest as tightness at the tempo-mandibular joint, causing discomfort in the jaw with possible headaches.

Classically, according to Chapter 13 of the *Ling Shu*, symptoms and signs of the San Jiao Sinew channel are said to be worse during the late Summer (July), and simply include stiffness, pain and/or spasm along the channel trajectory.

Arm Yang Ming (Large Intestine) Sinew channel

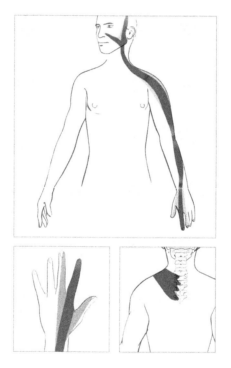

According to Chapter 13 of the *Ling Shu*, the sinews of the Large Intestine channel start from the index finger and bind at the wrist. They then run along the arm and bind at the lateral side of the elbow. From here, they ascend along the medial side of the arm and bind at the Jian Yu (LI-15). A branch circles around the scapula and attaches to the spine. The straight branch runs from Jian Yu (LI-15) to the neck. Another branch ascends to the cheek and binds at the side of the nose. Another straight branch runs upward to emerge in front of the Small Intestine Sinew channel, ascends to the corner of the forehead, connects with the head and descends to the right mandible.

Western anatomy associated with the Large Intestine Sinew channel

The major muscles and tendons, in regards to Western anatomy, that are associated with the trajectory and activation of the Large Intestine Sinew Channel are as follows (listed in alphabetical order):

- Abductor pollicis longus
- Brachiradialis
- Dorsal interosseous
- Extensor carpi radialis longus
- Extensor digitorum superficialis
- Extensor pollicis brevis, longus
- Infrahyoids
- Infraspinatus
- Lateral deltoid
- Levator scapulae
- Platysma
- Rhomboids, major, minor
- Sternocleidomastoid
- Supinator
- Suprahyoids
- Supraspinatus
- Trapezius
- Triceps (lateral head)

Note: The actual muscles and tendons associated with the Large Intestine Sinew channel may indeed be more extensive than the list above. Due to the complex nature of functional movement, it is difficult to determine exactly which individual muscles and tendons are involved with each specific Sinew channel. The above list of muscles and tendons is based on clinical experience and observation in addition to anatomical understanding and modern research on the musculoskeletal system, and includes only major components of the musculoskeletal system. It is also important to note that some muscles and tendons will indeed be associated with multiple Sinew channels.

Mechanisms and movements of the Large Intestine Sinew channel

The Large Intestine Sinew channel is the arm aspect of the Yang Ming channel. As mentioned previously in regards to the Stomach Sinew channel, the Yang Ming channels are located on the anterior aspect of the body when stood in a neutral position, and are mainly related to our ability to brace ourselves and to bear weight, in addition to reaching out in front of us.

Large Intestine Sinew channel

The movement of the Large Intestine can be seen by lifting the arms in front in order to push an object away, but also to bring objects towards us.

The Large Intestine Sinew channel is unique among the Sinew channels in a way that it has both a Yin and Yang movement. It is the Large Intestine Sinew channel that gives the ability to lift the arms in front in order to push an object away, but also to bring objects towards us. It is essentially the Sinew channel that acts as the interaction between the outward movement of Yang and the pulling inward movement of Yin (which is thought to be why the Large Intestine Sinew channel is the final Yang Sinew channel before the Wei Qi circulates through the Yin Sinew channels). What's more, due to the channel ascending the front of the neck and passing over the head, the Large Intestine Sinew channel assists in turning the head.

Symptoms and signs of the Large Intestine Sinew channel

Symptoms and signs of the Large Intestine Sinew channel are classically said to be worse during early Summer (May), and include the inability to reach out without discomfort or pain. The patient will feel week when using the arms to brace themselves, and will not be able to hold any weight out in front of them. Due to the trajectory ascending the neck and passing over the head, difficulty in turning the head or bracing the neck may occur when there is tension in upper aspects of the Sinew channel. According to Chapter 13 of the *Ling Shu*, there may be muscle stiffness, pain and/or spasms experienced in the areas that the channel passes, and an inability to raise the shoulders and difficulty in turning the neck.

Leg Tai Yin (Spleen) Sinew channel

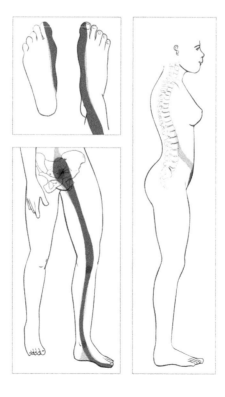

According to Chapter 13 of the *Ling Shu*, the sinews of the Spleen channel start at the medial side of the big toe and bind at the medial malleolus. A straight branch connects with the medial side of the knee, runs along the medial side of the thigh, binds at the hip and converges around the external genitalia. From here, a branch ascends to the abdomen and binds at the navel. Travelling within the abdomen, it binds at the ribs and disperses in the chest. An internal branch connects to the spine.

Western anatomy associated with the Spleen Sinew channel

The major muscles and tendons, in regards to Western anatomy, that are associated with the trajectory and activation of the Spleen Sinew Channel are as follows (listed in alphabetical order):

- Abductor brevis, hallucis
- Adductor longus, magnus
- External obliques
- Flexor digitorum longus
- Flexor hallucis longus
- Iliacus
- Intercostals
- Pectineus
- Psoas
- Sartorius
- Serratus anterior
- Tendon of the quadriceps femoris
- Tibialis posterior
- Vastus medialis

Note: The actual muscles and tendons associated with the Spleen Sinew channel may indeed be more extensive than the list above. Due to the complex nature of functional movement, it is difficult to determine exactly which individual muscles and tendons are involved with each specific Sinew channel. The above list of muscles and tendons is based on clinical experience and observation in addition to anatomical understanding and modern research on the musculoskeletal system, and includes only major components of the musculoskeletal system. It is also important to note that some muscles and tendons will indeed be associated with multiple Sinew channels.

Mechanisms and movements of the Spleen Sinew channel

The Tai Yin Sinew channels are classed as the first of the Yin channels, and therefore considered to be the most exterior of the Yin channels. They are located on the medial aspects of the limbs and the torso, and are involved in the initial yet simple inward movement of the limbs towards the body. The Spleen Sinew channel is the leg aspect of the Tai Yin Sinew channel.

Spleen Sinew channel

The movement of the Spleen Sinew channel involves bringing the lower limbs inwards towards the body, and can be seen as we go to sit down by bending at the waist and lowering ourselves steadily into a chair, or by lifting our knees up to our torso. It is the Spleen Sinew channel that also gives structure and support to the arches of the feet and stability to the medial aspect of the ankle.

Symptoms and signs of the Spleen Sinew channel

Due to the nature of the inward movement of the Spleen Sinew channel, when it has been affected by injury or the invasion of pathogens, the patient will find it difficult to make movements towards the centre of the body. This may manifest as difficulty in bringing the knees up to the abdomen, or being unable to lower themselves into a chair in a controlled manner or without discomfort (especially in the hips). Issues with the Spleen Sinew channel may also cause dropped arches, instability of the ankles and discomfort along the inner thigh and hip.

Classically, symptoms and signs of the Spleen Sinew channel were said to be worse during mid-Autumn (September). According to Chapter 13 of the *Ling Shu*, diseases involving the Spleen Sinew channel include stiffness of the big toe, pain around the medial malleolus, pain in the bone medial to the knee, hip pain due to contraction of the inner thigh, colic-type pain in the external genitalia and referred pain from the naval to the chest and spine (in accordance with the channel trajectory).

Arm Tai Yin (Lung) Sinew channel

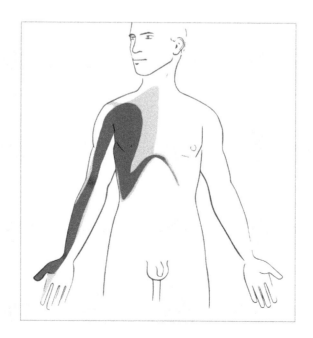

According to Chapter 13 of the *Ling Shu*, the sinews of the Lung channel start at the top of the thumb, run upward along the finger and bind at the thenar eminence. Along the lateral side of the Cun Kou pulse position, they run upward along the arm and bind at the elbow. From here, the channel ascends along the medial side of the arm, enters the axilla, emerges from the supraclavicular fossa and binds anteriorly to Jian Yu (LI-15). Proceeding upward, the channel binds at the supraclavicular fossa in the upper and the chest in the lower. It then spreads through the diaphragm, joins with Pericardium Sinew channel below the diaphragm and reaches the hypochondrium.

Western anatomy associated with the Lung Sinew channel

The major muscles and tendons, in regards to Western anatomy, that are associated with the trajectory and activation of the Lung Sinew Channel are as follows (listed in alphabetical order):

- Anterior deltoid
- Biceps brachii
- Brachialis
- Brachiradialis
- Diaphragm
- External/internal intercostals
- Flexor carpi radialis
- Flexor digitorum superficialis
- Flexor pollicis longus
- Major thenar eminence
- Pectorals, major, minor
- Pronators
- Subclavicus
- Supinators

Note: The actual muscles and tendons associated with the Lung Sinew channel may indeed be more extensive than the list above. Due to the complex nature of functional movement, it is difficult to determine exactly which individual muscles and tendons are involved with each specific Sinew channel. The above list of muscles and tendons is based on clinical experience and observation in addition to anatomical understanding and modern research on the musculoskeletal system, and includes only major components of the musculoskeletal system. It is also important to note that some muscles and tendons will indeed be associated with multiple Sinew channels.

Mechanisms and movements of the Lung Sinew channel

The Lung Sinew channel is the arm aspect of the Tai Yin Sinew channel. As mentioned above, the Tai Yin Sinew channels are classed as the first of the Yin channels, and therefore considered to be the most exterior of the Yin channels. They are located on the medial aspects of the limbs and the torso, and are involved in the initial yet simple inward movement of the limbs towards the body.

The Lung Sinew channel is also important for the breath. This is not only because the channel helps to open up the chest, as mentioned above, but also due to the fact that the channel acts on and engages both the intercostals, and the diaphragm. Both are important sets of muscles for the regulation of breath.

Lung Sinew channel

The movement of the Lung Sinew channel involves bringing the upper limbs inwards towards the torso, and can be seen by bringing the hand towards the shoulder by bending at the elbow. Strength in the Lung Sinew channel also helps to support good posture and alignment of the shoulders, and keeps the chest open by preventing a collapse of the shoulders and chest.

Symptoms and signs of the Lung Sinew channel

Injury or dysfunction of the Lung Sinew channel most commonly manifests as pain during parts of the breath due to the connection to the intercostal muscles and the diaphragm. Pain can also manifest at the delto-pectoral triangle during a deep inward breath, especially when the posture of the shoulders and chest has collapsed. Pain may also radiate from the shoulder down the arm along the bicep, or into the chest to the pectoral muscles.

Signs and symptoms of the Lung Sinew channel are classically said to become worse during mid-Winter (December). According to Chapter 13 of the *Ling Shu*, diseases of the Lung Sinew channel include stiffness, pain and/or spasms within the regions through which the sinews pass, Xi Ben disease (pain caused by excess Lung Qi stagnated below the hypochondrium, causing panting and painful breathing) and painful spasms of the diaphragm.

Leg Shao Yin (Kidney) Sinew channel

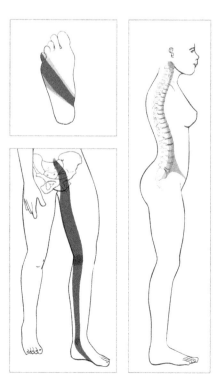

According to Chapter 13 of the *Ling Shu*, the Sinews of the Kidney channel start from the inferior side of the little toe, meet with the Sinews of Spleen channel, obliquely run below the medial malleolus and bind at the heel. Converging with the Bladder Sinew channel, they bind at the lower and medial side of the knee. The channel then meets with the Spleen Sinew channel to run upward along the medial side of the thigh and binds at the external genitalia. From here, the channel ascends from inside of the gluteal muscles and along the anterior spine to the neck, binds at the occipital bone and convergences with the Bladder Sinew channel.

Western anatomy associated with the Kidney Sinew channel

The major muscles and tendons, in regards to Western anatomy, that are associated with the trajectory and activation of the Kidney Sinew Channel are as follows (listed in alphabetical order):

- Adductor brevis, longus, magnus
- Anterior longitudinal ligament (of the spine)
- Diaphragm
- Flexor digitorum brevis, longus
- Flexor hallucis longus
- Gastrocnemius
- Gracilis
- Iliacus
- Longus capitis, colli
- Pectineus
- Plantar
- Psoas
- Pyramidalis
- Rectus abdominis
- Rectus capitis anterior, lateralis
- Sartorius
- Semimembranosus
- Semitendinosus
- Soleus
- Tibialis posterior
- Vastus medialis

Note: The actual muscles and tendons associated with the Kidney Sinew channel may indeed be more extensive than the list above. Due to the complex nature of functional movement, it is difficult to determine exactly which individual muscles and tendons are involved with each specific Sinew channel. The above list of muscles and tendons is based on clinical experience and observation in addition to anatomical understanding and modern research on the musculoskeletal system, and includes only major components of the musculoskeletal system. It is also important to note that some muscles and tendons will indeed be associated with multiple Sinew channels.

Mechanisms and movements of the Kidney Sinew channel

The Kidney Sinew channel is the leg aspect of the Shao Yin Sinew channel. Chapter 6 of the *Su Wen* states that the Shao Yin acts as the internal pivot (Shao Yin Wei Shu, 少阴为枢). Whereas the Shao Yang Sinew channels act as the external pivot (therefore lateral rotation), the Shao Yin Sinew channels help to act as an internal pivot, and therefore govern medial or inward rotation. The Shao Yin Sinew channels also assist the Shao Yang Sinew channels in rotation of the torso, and do so from within the core of the body (notice that the Kidney Sinew channel travels deep within the body and ascends upwards within the spine).

Kidney Sinew channel

The movement of the Kidney Sinew channel can be clearly seen during inward rotation of the hips, in a movement that in Chinese Arts is called 'closing the Kua'. In certain Chinese Arts, such as Qi Gong and TaiJi, the movement of 'closing the Kua' involves activation and engagement of the Kidney Sinew channels. When the Kidney Sinew channels are engaged too much, for instance, in a pigeon-toed stance, this causes tension in the lumbar aspect of the Kidney Sinew channel and is actually thought to close the fascia around the Ming Men area.

As the Kidney Sinew channel ascends and stabilises the Spine, it also helps in flexibility and mobility of the spine in all directions. The Kidney Sinew channel helps to stabilise the knees, especially the medial aspect of the knees, and assists the Spleen Sinew channel in stabilising the ankle through the medial aspect of the Achilles tendon.

Symptoms and signs of the Kidney Sinew channel

When the Kidney Sinew channels are injured, there will be discomfort and inflexibility of the spine due to anterior longitudinal ligament of the spine. This would be in movements of all directions, most notably in flexion, extension and rotation, and be felt deep within the body along the whole spine. Due to the Kidney Sinew channel stabilising the knees, weak knees with discomfort is also a sign of a Kidney Sinew channel pathology, as is being 'knock-kneed' or having inward-turning feet.

Symptoms and signs of the Kidney Sinew channel are quite unique due to the possibility of injury to the sinews also causing epilepsy and convulsions. This is again due to the channel passing up through the inside of the spine and into the cranium, affecting the nervous system. Additionally, occipital headaches are a sign of dysfunction of the Kidney Sinew channel due to it attaching to the occipital bone. This would manifest alongside tightness in the spine, and become exacerbated when the spine and neck are in flexion. Patients will commonly feel an uncomfortable pull in their lower back whilst putting their chin on their chest.

Signs and symptoms of the Kidney Sinew channel are classically said to become worse during Early-Autumn (August). According to Chapter 13 of the *Ling Shu*, diseases of the Kidney Sinew channel may include spasm and pain along the regions through which the sinews pass, epilepsy and convulsions, and an inability to look down due to tightness along the back aspect of the channel or to look up due to tightness along the front aspect of the channel.

Arm Shao Yin (Heart) Sinew channel

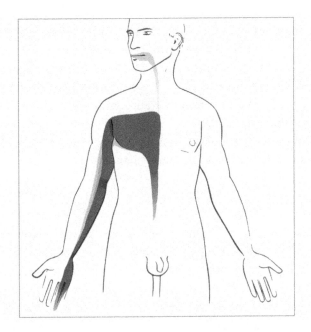

According to Chapter 13 of the *Ling Shu*, the sinews of the Heart channel start from the medial side of the little finger. From here, the channel runs upward to bind at the medial side of the elbow. The channel then ascends to the axilla, joins the Lung Sinew channel in the breast region and binds in the chest. The channel then runs downward across the diaphragm to connect with the navel.

Western anatomy associated with the Heart Sinew channel

The major muscles and tendons, in regards to Western anatomy, that are associated with the trajectory and activation of the Heart Sinew Channel are as follows (listed in alphabetical order):

- Abductor digiti minimi
- Biceps brachii
- Diaphragm
- Flexor carpi ulnaris, radialis

- Flexor digiti minimi brevis
- Flexor digitorum profundus, superficialis
- Intercostals
- Linea alba
- Lumbricals
- Opponens digiti minimi

- Palmaris brevis, longus
- Palmer interosseous
- Pectorals, major, minor
- Pronator quadratus, teres
- Rectus abdominis
- Transverse thoracis
- Triceps brachii (medial head)

Note: The actual muscles and tendons associated with the Heart Sinew channel may indeed be more extensive than the list above. Due to the complex nature of functional movement, it is difficult to determine exactly which individual muscles and tendons are involved with each specific Sinew channel. The above list of muscles and tendons is based on clinical experience and observation in addition to anatomical understanding and modern research on the musculoskeletal system, and includes only major components of the musculoskeletal system. It is also important to note that some muscles and tendons will indeed be associated with multiple Sinew channels.

Mechanisms and movements of the Heart Sinew channel

Whereas the Shao Yang Sinew channels act as the external pivot (therefore lateral rotation), the Shao Yin Sinew channels are sometimes considered to act as the internal pivot, and therefore govern medial rotation. The Heart Sinew channel is the arm aspect of the Shao Yin Sinew channel, and therefore governs internal rotation of the arms. In regards to the upper limbs, the Heart Sinew channel governs the complex movement of rotation and flexion. This movement can be seen, for example, when pouring a kettle of water, or bringing a cup towards the mouth and drinking.

Heart Sinew channel

The movement of the Heart Sinew channel can be seen, for example, when pouring a kettle of water, or bringing a cup towards the mouth and drinking. It can also be seen when putting your 'hand on your heart' or bringing someone closer in for a hug.

The Heart Sinew channel also has an internal connection up towards the root of the tongue and connects with the corners of the mouth, allowing free movement of the tongue and the ability to smile. It is said that smiling engages the tissues around the Heart and opens up the spaces around it.

Symptoms and signs of the Heart Sinew channel

When there is injury to the Heart Sinew channel, there will be pain at the elbow that is made worse by flexion and rotation. This commonly presents as golfer's elbow (medial epicondylitis). There may also be chest discomfort that spreads to the diaphragm, and a disliking of talking or difficulty speaking fluidly.

Signs and symptoms of the Heart Sinew channel are classically said to become worse during Late-Winter (January). According to Chapter 13 of the *Ling Shu*, diseases of the Heart Sinew channel simply include stiffness, pain and/or spasm of the regions through which the channel passes.

Leg Jue Yin (Liver) Sinew channel

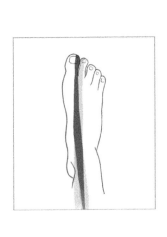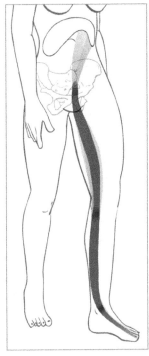

According to Chapter 13 of the *Ling Shu*, the sinews of the Liver channel start at the big toe and bind anteriorly to the medial malleolus. From here, the channel runs upward along the leg and binds at the medial side of the tibia. The channel then ascends along the medial side of the thigh, binds at the external genitalia and connects with other tendons.

Western anatomy associated with the Liver Sinew channel

The major muscles and tendons, in regards to Western anatomy, that are associated with the trajectory and activation of the Liver Sinew Channel are as follows (listed in alphabetical order):

- Adductor brevis
- Adductor longus
- Adductor magnus
- Diaphragm
- Dorsal interosseous
- Extensor hallucis brevis
- Gastrocnemius
- Gracilis
- Iliacus
- Pectineus
- Psoas major
- Pyramidalis
- Rectus abdominis
- Sartorius
- Soleus
- Vastus medialis

Note: The actual muscles and tendons associated with the Liver Sinew channel may indeed be more extensive than the list above. Due to the complex nature of functional movement, it is difficult to determine exactly which individual muscles and tendons are involved with each specific Sinew channel. The above list of muscles and tendons is based on clinical experience and observation in addition to anatomical understanding and modern research on the musculoskeletal system, and includes only major components of the musculoskeletal system. It is also important to note that some muscles and tendons will indeed be associated with multiple Sinew channels.

Mechanisms and movements of the Liver Sinew channel

The Jue Yin Sinew channels are mainly responsible for the movement of adduction, in addition to giving the ability to hold and support the body whilst relaxing in a lying-down position. The Jue Yin channels are also in control of the finer motor movements, which is why there can be a tremor or incoordination when the Jue Yin channels become dysfunctional. The Liver Sinew channel, which is the foot aspect of Jue Yin, is specifically responsible for adduction of the hip and contraction of both the male and female genitals during arousal.

Liver Sinew channel

The movement of the Liver Sinew channel can be seen by the smooth, fine motor movements of the limbs that originate from the torso (as opposed to the limbs acting as isolated levers), in addition to adducting the legs and contracting the genitals.

The Liver Sinew channel, along with the Pericardium Sinew channel, is also responsible for the finer motor movements of the limbs, therefore giving the ability to make smooth and coordinated movements. This is reflected in the Liver function of maintaining the smooth flow of Qi.

Symptoms and signs of the Liver Sinew channel

When there is injury to the Liver Sinew channel, there may be pain, discomfort and/ or weakness of the leg whilst performing adduction. Due to the connection to the diaphragm, there may also be difficulty breathing that will manifest in the outward breath. Liver Sinew channel disorders can also create jerky movements with sudden spasm or tremor whilst attempting to make smaller and finer movements. In extreme circumstances, there can be complete cessation of movement or paralysis, as the internal connective tissues cannot engage sufficiently, and the Vital Substances cannot circulate to the extremities.

Signs and symptoms of the Liver Sinew channel are classically said to become worse during Late-Autumn (October). According to Chapter 13 of the *Ling Shu*, diseases that affect the Liver Sinew channel may include stiffness of the big toe, pain to the anterior of the medial malleolus that runs upwards along the medial side of the tibia, or pain along the medial aspect of the thigh that radiates to the external genitalia and causes dysfunction. Dysfunction of the Liver Sinew channel may also give rise to erectile dysfunction that is made worse by excessive sexual activity.

Arm Jue Yin (Pericardium) Sinew channel

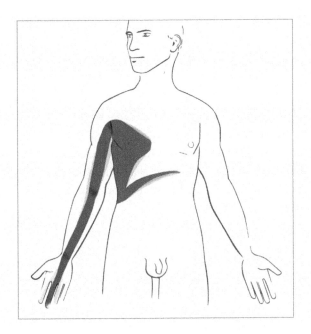

According to Chapter 13 of the *Ling Shu*, the sinews of the Pericardium channel start at the middle finger, run parallel to the Lung Sinew channel, and bind at the medial side of the elbow. From here, the channel ascends along the medial aspect of the arm, binds below the axilla where it then spreads at the front and back of the ribs. Its branch enters the axilla, spreads in the chest and binds at the arm.

Western anatomy associated with the Pericardium Sinew channel

The major muscles and tendons, in regards to Western anatomy, that are associated with the trajectory and activation of the Pericardium Sinew channel are as follows (listed in alphabetical order):

- Biceps brachii
- Brachialis
- Diaphragm
- Flexor carpi radialis
- Flexor digitorum superficialis
- Intercostals
- Lumbricals
- Palmaris brevis
- Palmar interosseous
- Palmaris longus
- Pectorals (major and minor)
- Pronators
- Transversus thoracis

Note: The actual muscles and tendons associated with the Pericardium Sinew channel may indeed be more extensive than the list above. Due to the complex nature of functional movement, it is difficult to determine exactly which individual muscles and tendons are involved with each specific Sinew channel. The above list of muscles and tendons is based on clinical experience and observation in addition to anatomical understanding and modern research on the musculoskeletal system, and includes only major components of the musculoskeletal system. It is also important to note that some muscles and tendons will indeed be associated with multiple Sinew channels.

Mechanisms and movements of the Pericardium Sinew channel

The Jue Yin Sinew channels in general are responsible for the movement of adduction, in addition to giving the ability to hold and support the body whilst relaxing in a lying-down, relaxed position. The Jue Yin channels are also in control of the finer motor movements, which is why there can be a tremor and incoordination when the Jue Yin channels become dysfunctional.

Pericardium Sinew channel

The movement of the Pericardium Sinew channel can be seen by clenching a fist and also adducting the arm. The Pericardium Sinew Channel is also responsible for supporting the movement of the diaphragm and opening the chest.

The Pericardium Sinew channel, which is the hand aspect of Jue Yin, is specifically responsible for adduction of the upper limbs, in addition to clenching a fist. The Pericardium Sinew channel, similar to the Liver Sinew channel in regards to the lower limbs and trunk, is also responsible for the finer motor movements of the upper limbs and trunk, therefore giving the ability to make smooth and coordinated movements, including with our breathing. What's more, the Pericardium Sinew channel also has a key responsibility for the internal connective tissues that engage the diaphragm and open the chest, which in turn helps the circulation of the Vital Substances within the body and helps to guide them to and through the extremities. This is why opening the Pericardium channel (and the point P-8, Lao Gong) is such a major aspect of energetic practices such as Qi Gong and Dao Yin.

Symptoms and signs of the Pericardium Sinew channel

When there is injury to the Pericardium Sinew channel, there may be pain, discomfort and/or weakness of the ribs and chest whilst performing adduction with the arm. Again, like the Liver Sinew channel, there may also be difficulty breathing due to the connection to the diaphragm. Pericardium Sinew channel disorders can also create jerky movements with breathing and use of the upper limbs. In extreme circumstances, there can be complete cessation of movement or paralysis, as the internal connective tissues of the chest and diaphragm cannot engage sufficiently, and the Vital Substances cannot circulate to the extremities.

Signs and symptoms of the Pericardium Sinew channel are classically said to become worse during Early-Winter (November). According to Chapter 13 of the *Ling Shu*, diseases of the Pericardium Sinew channel include stiffness, pain and/or spasm of the regions through which the channel passes, and pain caused by stagnation of Qi accumulating below the diaphragm.

DIAGNOSTICS OF TUI NA

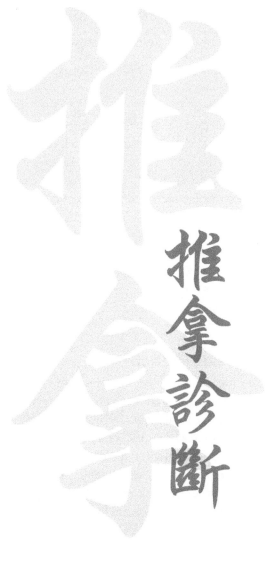

Chapter 4

Diagnostics of Tui Na

The contents of this section cover a relatively brief overview of Chinese Medicine diagnostics, with a major focus on the assessment and diagnosis of the Sinew channels, due to the external nature of Tui Na as a therapy. These include the following methods:

- Assessment of the Sinew channels through palpation, observation and inquiry.

- Assessment of the Sinew channels through movement.

- Assessment of the Sinew channels through strength and engagement.

- Special examinations.

Tui Na is, of course, a whole medical system, and can indeed be used to successfully treat both non-musculoskeletal conditions and internal diseases. For assessment and diagnostic methods within the field of internal medicine, it is vitally important that a full Chinese Medicine diagnosis aimed at the Zang Fu (organs) and the Primary channels is made in order to effectively and safely treat correctly. This would include the in-depth use of palpation (including pulse), observation (including tongue), listening and smelling, and inquiry methods of diagnosis, and analysing these methods using the Eight Principles and pattern syndrome differentiation. To include all of these diagnostic methods into this book would be too much, therefore I felt it best to focus on Tui Na specific assessment and diagnostic methods with a bias toward musculoskeletal conditions and the Sinew channels.

A brief note on disease location

When we think of pain from a Chinese Medicine point of view, we think of Qi (氣) stagnation (explained later in this section) which is essentially a blockage. Many practitioners simply treat the site of the stagnation. Whilst logically this makes sense, that is, when someone is experiencing back pain we treat the back, we would most likely be missing the bigger picture. Qi stagnation is just a symptom, and the location where the patient feels the Qi stagnate often has nothing to do with the problem, unless there has been some direct trauma to that area. Pain can be one of the most misleading things to treat for this reason!

When pain has developed seemingly out of the blue, there is often an underlying Yin pattern in the Sinew channels (such as underactivity or hypotonicity), a Yang pattern in the Sinew channels (such as hyperactivity or hypertonicity), or a dysfunction somewhere along the Sinew channel system. This is why, as Tui Na practitioners, we must assess all Sinew channels that run through the area of dysfunction through palpation, observation and by testing their strength and engagement. This enables us to diagnose why the Qi stagnation or pain is happening, as essentially if we don't correctly diagnose, then we are just guessing.

The importance of the Diaphragm and breathing

The importance of breathing cannot be underestimated when dealing with conditions such as Qi stagnation and overall health. From a Chinese Medicine perspective, the only two ways we acquire Qi is from the food that we eat and the air that we *breathe*. So breathing is very important for moving Qi around the body and improving overall health. If we are not breathing properly, how can the body circulate Qi effectively?

As human beings, we breathe roughly between 20,000–25,000 times a day. If our breathing becomes dysfunctional, this can wreak havoc on the whole body. Ideally when we breathe, we should draw our breath down to below our Diaphragm and into our lower Dan Tian (丹田) – this is known as connecting the Lungs to the Kidneys. Our breath should also expand in the 360-degree cylinder through the front and the back, encompassing the Dai Mai (帶脈, Girdling vessel). A healthy Dai Mai has a large influence on the healthy circulation of Qi and Blood, particularly within the lower Jiao. In Chinese Medicine, the Lungs are considered to be the highest of the Zang organs, and therefore descend and disperse the Qi. The Diaphragm sits just under the Lungs, and when breathing becomes dysfunctional, the Diaphragm becomes stuck or simply doesn't move well. This prevents the descending and dispersing of the Qi. As the Lungs are essentially big bellows, if they are unable to expand properly, there will be pressure problems within the body (known as intra-abdominal pressure issues), resulting in a stagnation of Qi.

The Diaphragm is not only important for being responsible for assisting the Lungs in moving Qi by descending and dispersing, but also because it connects to various other parts of the body. It also attaches to the roof of the mouth – this is why, in Taiji (太极) and Qi Gong (氣功), practitioners will press their tongue onto the roof of the mouth in order to make a connection between the Ren Mai and Du Mai. Doing so creates a fascial and neural connection with the Diaphragm and the circulation of Vital Substances that it helps with. This also explains why one of the core foundations and practices of Taiji and Qi Gong is diaphragmatic breathing. The Diaphragm also connects with the spine, which again is hugely important within energetic practices such as Taiji and Qi Gong for the transfer of power and circulation of the Vital Substances.

The Diaphragm also attaches to both the front and the back of the body. If the Lung and Diaphragm functions are impaired, it can cause pain or discomfort to the back and front. The Diaphragm also has fascial connections to the pelvis, and in particular, the psoas muscle (part of the Stomach, Spleen, Liver and Kidney Sinew channels). If Lung and Diaphragm functions are impaired, and the ability to move Qi around the body is vastly reduced, this will, of course, affect the channel system, particularly in the lower Jiao, causing stagnation or even deficiency of the organs and tissues within the pelvic region.

Lastly, the Lungs in Chinese Medicine are responsible for water metabolism and dissemination of the Body Fluids, and do so with the help of diaphragmatic breathing. This is because the Diaphragm is one of the main lymphatic pumps of the body. Should the Diaphragm not pump effectively enough, the Body Fluids will stagnate and again, cause pain and discomfort. Your body is essentially bathed in lymph – when we talk about nourishing the Yin and Body Fluids within Chinese Medicine, the lymphatic system can be considered as one of those key components. The Lungs connect to the skin, and the lymphatic system sits just beneath the skin. If the body is injured or in need of repair, the lymphatic system is involved by helping to draw 'cellular waste' away from the injury site. For example, DOMS (delayed onset muscle soreness) is a result of inflammation within the fascia, muscles and connective tissues, and the lymphatic system is responsible for getting rid of this inflammation. If the body is unable to do this, for instance, due to a dysfunction of the Diaphragm, the DOMS will feel worse and last for longer. This is also a key reason why some people will wake up in the morning with the feeling of achiness all over until they begin to move. This is often due to the breathing being too shallow during sleep, and the Diaphragm has not been active enough to help circulate the fluids around the body, thus causing stagnation. If the Diaphragm doesn't move properly, it also doesn't move and 'massage' the Zang Fu organs, causing them to suffer from stagnation and become dysfunctional as well. As a result, this will cause a wide range of problems, mostly due to stagnation (discussed below). In addition to stagnation, a dysfunctional Diaphragm movement can cause Qi deficiency due to the lack of Qi and Blood circulation, essentially causing malnourishment of various parts of the body.

Understanding pain in Chinese Medicine

Before getting into assessment methods and diagnosis, it is first important to understand the nature of pain, and what pain is in regards to Chinese Medicine. All pain, no matter where or what the cause is, has an element of Qi stagnation. Basically, pain = stagnation. It is the stagnation of Qi that is telling the body that something is not right, causing the body to give out a warning by giving the sensation of pain. What we need to do is simply get things moving as they should be again.

In Chinese Medicine, we have what are called the Liu Yu (六郁, Six Stagnations). The Six Stagnations are Qi stagnation, Blood stagnation (also known as Blood stasis), Phlegm stagnation, Damp stagnation, Fire stagnation and Food stagnation. Each type of stagnation begins with the stagnation of Qi, which, if left untreated, can lead on to the stagnation of physical substances such as Blood, Phlegm, Damp or Food, or create Heat as a result of constriction and lack of movement (much like friction generates Heat), giving rise to what is known as Fire stagnation. Therefore, treatment of any stagnation type should focus on moving and resolving Qi stagnation first and foremost. All types of stagnation will cause discomfort and pain somewhere within the body, and it is important to identify which type of stagnation is present. It should be noted that, classically, Cold stagnation was also discussed as one of the stagnation types; however, in this context it would be a cause of stagnation rather than a substance that has stagnated. Stagnation due to Cold is discussed below, when covering the 'nature of pain'.

Qi (氣) stagnation

Qi stagnation essentially means that the Qi has simply become 'stuck' and the circulation is impeded – it is not flowing as it should. Note that when Qi 'stagnates', it does not actually ever stop; it simply slows down and becomes constricted. (However, when physical substances such as Blood, Phlegm or Food become stagnated, they often do actually come to a stop and do not move.) If the Qi has become stagnated, in addition to causing pain or discomfort, over time it will also cause other substances to become stagnated. This is because it is the Qi that moves the Blood and Body Fluids, and also gives the ability to move food through the digestive tract.

Stagnation means pain or discomfort, and all pain within the body is due to a stagnation of the Qi, whether directly or not. Many factors can cause the Qi to stagnate, such as pathogenic factors, diet and lifestyle, physical trauma and even emotional trauma. If these causes are not kept in check, they may cause obstruction and/or constriction within the channels that lead to pain and discomfort. Some factors cause immediate pain, such as physical trauma, whereas others will cause pain over a period of time, such as emotional trauma or diet and lifestyle. Whatever the cause is, it must be identified so that it does not happen again, once we resolve the stagnation.

Blood (血, Xue) stagnation (or stasis)

Stagnation of Blood (also known as Blood stasis) can be identified by a clearly fixed, stabbing pain. The pain may also become worse during the night – this is due to Blood being a Yin substance, and substances flow with less force at night because of the lack of motive force from Yang. There may also be the appearance of bruising along the Sinew channels, or purple areas on the tongue.

Phlegm (痰, Tan) stagnation

Stagnation that is caused by the build-up of Phlegm in the channels will cause a distending yet dull pain, and will be accompanied by nodules, lumps or bumps in the channels that are clearly palpable. There will also be a restrictive feeling within the channels to both the patient and practitioner.

Damp (濕, Shi) stagnation

Stagnation that is caused by Damp will often result in the feeling of heavy limbs and a dull aching pain. The skin in areas that are affected by Damp stagnation may appear slightly yellow, and feel slightly swollen or puffy compared to other parts of the body.

Movement of the affected Sinew channel(s) will also be sluggish and lethargic, and some patients may describe that they feel 'sick in the limb'. More information on Damp type pain can be found below, when discussing the 'nature of pain'.

Fire (火, Huo) stagnation

Fire stagnation is often accompanied by a feeling of warmth to the area of stagnation, in addition to an aversion to Heat. The affected channels may also appear red, and feel warm to touch compared to other parts of the body.

Food (食, Shi) stagnation

Stagnation that is caused by food is usually felt within the Stomach and/or the Small Intestine. The abdomen will often be bloated, with a distending type pain. Patients will also develop a low appetite as the body is aware that the food previously eaten has not yet been fully digested, and there may also be signs of constipation.

The nature of pain

When we are presented with injuries or conditions showing symptoms of pain, we want to know about the nature of the pain, that is, what the patient's pain feels like. Different causes of pain will be experienced in different ways, and asking how the patient describes their pain in addition to palpating the areas of pain or discomfort can help us to identify the nature of the pain and what is involved with causing them pain.

Types of pain can be separated into two main categories – of deficiency (虚, Xu) and excess (实, Shi), with the latter being split further into the different types of excesses. These are discussed below.

Deficiency (虚, Xu) type pain

Within Chinese Medicine, when something is described as deficient (虚, Xu), it essentially means that something that should be there is now lacking or not functioning properly to its full potential. This commonly refers to the Vital Substances, such as Qi, Blood, Body Fluids, Yin or Yang.

Deficiency commonly causes stagnation of Qi or Qi and Blood, because the mechanisms of keeping a steady flow of Qi and Blood are no longer working in one way or another. For instance, if there is a Qi or Yang deficiency, there will not be enough of a 'motive force' in order to keep a healthy circulation of Qi and Blood within the vessels, as it is said that 'Qi that moves Blood'. Conversely, due to the fact that 'Blood carries Qi', if there is a Yin or Blood deficiency, there will not be enough of a material foundation to help 'carry' the Qi, therefore causing it to stagnate.

Deficiency type pain is characterised by pain that is alleviated with applied pressure and/or pain that is made worse with movement or exertion. The pulse is likely to feel weak and feeble, due to there being a lack of one or more of the vital substances.

Signs and symptoms of deficiency (虛, Xu) type pain

- Pain that is alleviated by applying pressure.

- Pain that is made worse with movement and exertion.

- Weak pulse.

Excess (实, Shi) type pain

Within Chinese Medicine, when something is described as excess, it essentially means that something is there that shouldn't be. This most commonly refers to the presence of pathogenic Qi, also known as Xie Qi (邪氣). In regards to pain, the presence of pathogenic Qi is causing an obstruction within the channels, causing a stagnation of Qi.

If the pain that is experienced by the patient is of an excess type, it will typically feel worse if pressure is applied, and also feel worse if exposed to the type of pathogen that is causing the pain (such as a Cold type pain feeling worse in the Cold). The pulse is likely to feel excessively strong and full. Other symptoms of excess type pain will depend on the type of pathogen that is causing the obstruction and pain, and these are discussed below.

Signs and symptoms of excess (实, Shi) type pain

- Pain that is made worse by applying pressure. Other symptoms also depend on which pathogen(s) is present.

- Strong or full pulse.

Wind (风, Feng) type pain

Wind, known as Feng (风) in Chinese, is the predominant Qi during the Spring season, but diseases caused by Wind may occur in any of the other seasons. Wind type pain is caused by excess Wind Qi causing contraction and tightening of the tendons and sinews. The resulting muscle stiffness and rigidity from the tissue contraction disrupts the flow of Qi and Blood through the Sinew channels, thus causing Qi stagnation and pain, in addition to restricted or unsmooth movements.

In the natural world, Wind blows in gusts, and Wind type conditions within Chinese Medicine are therefore characterised by unpredictability and sudden changes. Pain due to Wind tends be very Yang in nature – it changes in location (often from joint to joint), has sudden and rapid changes, and can also be sudden onset. Wind type pain is often referred to as 'wandering' pain because of these characteristics.

When taking the pulse, Wind type pain will manifest as a taut and wiry pulse at the positions of the corresponding channels. This is due to the Sinew channels becoming taut and having an effect on the Qi and Blood flowing through them.

Signs and symptoms of Wind (风, Feng) type pain

- Sudden pain that moves around (known as wandering pain).

- Sudden onset.

- Rapid change in symptoms.

- Stiffness and pain in the joints and rigidity of the muscles.

- Taut and wiry pulse.

Damp (湿, Shi) type pain

Damp is a classed as a Yin pathogen due to its heavy and downward moving actions. Damp is common in climates that are wet, such as areas close to rivers, or locations such as the north of the UK, where there is more rain and moisture in the air. It can also be caused by damp living conditions, or exposure to damp caused by sweat or exposure to water such as swimming. As Dampness is a Yin pathogen, it can easily obstruct the circulation of Qi due to its heavy, thick, viscous nature. It is also most likely to occur in the lower regions of the body, such as the knees and lower back.

Damp type pain is characterised by a dull ache that is often accompanied by a heavy sensation within the affected channel or region of the body. Some patients may complain of a 'discomfort' rather than a pain, and there will likely also be swelling within the local joints or along the channel causing stiffness. If there is Dampness within the Sinew channel causing the pain, the pulse corresponding to the channel that the pain is present in will likely be slippery.

Signs and symptoms of Damp (湿, Shi) type pain

- Dull ache type pain accompanied by a heavy sensation.

- Possible swelling at the site of injury.

- Made worse in damp and wet climates.

- Slippery pulse.

Cold (寒, Han) type pain

Cold, known as Han (寒) in Chinese, is a type of Qi that causes a slowing down and contraction of the body's mechanisms. It most commonly occurs in the Winter, but may also cause disease or injury at any other time of year if the climate or surroundings are cold enough. Cold type pain occurs due to stagnation as a consequence of restricted Qi and Blood flow resulting from the contraction of the vessels and surrounding body tissues. However, the body tissues do not contract so suddenly or quickly as they would with Wind, and do so slowly causing rigidity and stiffness. The lack of warmth and blood flow to the area can also cause the tissues to become 'brittle', making them more susceptible to injury or damage. Again, due to the contracting nature of Cold type Qi, injury or disease is typically confined to just one joint or localised area.

Cold type pain is characterised by a fixed, stabbing pain that may be cold to touch and have a possible pale or even cyanotic appearance to the skin in the local area. There may also be an aversion to Cold, and application of warmth will alleviate pain. Due to the nature of Cold type Qi causing slowness of movement and contraction of the vessels, the pulse at the positions of the corresponding channels will be slow and taut.

Signs and symptoms of Cold (寒, Han) type pain

- Cold, stabbing and fixed pain.

- Stiffness and rigidity with possible spasm.

- Feeling of cold at the injury site that is penetrating.

- Pale or cyanotic appearance to the localised area.

- Aversion to the cold.

- Slow, taut pulse.

Heat (热, Re) type pain

Heat type pain is not often caused by externally contracted Heat, but caused as a by-product of Wei Qi becoming stagnated at an injury site during the healing process, or by excessive internal heat caused by a deficiency of Yin. If it is due to the former, it will be acute.

Heat type pain is often severe, throbbing and can radiate along a channel. The area of the injury would often be red and hot to the touch, and can also appear swollen due to the heat causing expansion of the vessels and allowing more fluids into the area. Essentially, when an injury is referred to as being 'inflamed', this would come under the category of Heat type pain. Due to Heat type Qi causing hyperactivity, the pulse at the positions of the corresponding channels will be rapid and/or surging.

Signs and symptoms of Heat (热, Re) type pain

- Severe, radiating and/or throbbing pain.

- Feeling of warmth and redness at the site of injury.

- Aversion to warmth and Heat.

- Rapid or surging pulse.

Chapter 5

Assessment of the Sinew Channels through Observation, Inquiry and Palpation

Assessment of the Sinew channels is primarily done through visual observation, inquiry and palpation. Each method has its own strengths and weaknesses, and therefore all three methods of assessment are needed to guide and build a comprehensive diagnosis, therefore creating an effective treatment plan and prescription. Observation, inquiry and palpation form the basis of all other methods of assessment that are discussed later in this section, and require the practitioner to be alert at all times during both the consultation and the treatment, in addition to being able to multi-task whilst thinking laterally and spontaneously. The following covers a brief overview of each method of diagnosis, focusing on their use for assessing the Sinew channels from a Tui Na perspective.

Observation

When diagnosing disorders of the Sinew channels, it is important that we visually observe the patient and the Sinew channels in both a resting state and an active state. More detailed information on observing the Sinew channels in an active state can be found later in this section, within 'Assessment of the Sinew channels through movement' and 'Assessment of the Sinew channels through strength and engagement'.

Diagnosis by observation can be split into two main categories – general observations (which include posture, natural body movement and observation of the Shen, 神) and specific observations (which include swellings or enlargements, atrophies or weaknesses, colours and/or bruising, deformities and abnormalities and breathing patterns).

General observations

With diagnosis by observation, we are able to assess the patient from the moment we set eyes on them, perhaps even before they have entered the treatment room. Immediately, we are able to see their *natural* posture as well as their *natural* body movement. It is important that we observe these states in a natural way, as often the patient's movements and posture will alter as soon as they feel that they are being observed and assessed.

This is a subconscious action, and sometimes can't be helped. Observing the posture and body movement when the patient is unaware can help us see the true picture, and gives us a general understanding before the consultation has started.

Posture

When initially observing the patient's posture, we are looking at both the general constitution of the patient, in addition to deficiencies or excesses of specific Sinew channels. For example, if the patient appears to have a solid and sturdy posture, this demonstrates that the patient is healthy with a good constitution, and is more likely to suffer from excess (Shi, 实) type conditions. If the patient appears weak and feeble on the other hand, it demonstrates that the patient is likely to have a weak constitution, and is more likely to suffer from deficiency (Xu, 虚) type conditions. In regards to the Sinew channels, a strong upright posture may indicate that there is an excess in the Bladder Sinew channel, whereas a slumped posture with a concave chest could indicate that there is a weakness in the Lung Sinew channel.

More specific observations of the posture, such as curvatures of the spine and pelvic alignment, are discussed later, under 'Special examinations' in Chapter 7. A list of basic posture types can be found in the table below:

Posture type	Indication
Strong and sturdy	Healthy with a good constitution
Weak and feeble	Deficiency (Xu, 虚) type conditions
Tense or rigid	Excess (Shi, 实) Yang Qi or Liver Qi stagnation
Flaccid	Deficiency (Xu, 虚) type conditions
Strong, upright	Excess (Shi, 实) of the Bladder channel
Slumped, with a concave chest	Deficiency (Xu, 虚) of the Lung channel
Raised shoulders	Excess (Shi, 实) Yang Qi or Liver Yang Rising
Rounded shoulders	Excess (Shi, 实) of the Lung channel
Leg(s) rotating inwards	Excess (Shi, 实) of the Kidney channel or deficiency (Xu, 虚) of the Gall Bladder channel
Leg(s) rotating outwards	Excess (Shi, 实) of the Gall Bladder channel or deficiency (Xu, 虚) of the Kidney channel
Creased at the waist	Deficiency (Xu, 虚) of the Bladder or Stomach channel

Natural body movement

In addition to observing the patient's posture from the moment we see them, we are also able to observe the way that they move in a natural setting. We can see how they approach to greet us, how they enter the treatment room, how they are able to sit down on the chair and stand up again, and how easy or difficult it is for them to get on to the treatment couch. These natural movements are just as important as the ones seen when asked to perform specific actions during the assessment, as these movements are usually done subconsciously and without the thought of being assessed. Asking the patient to simply hang their coat up, for instance, is likely to give a different outcome to asking them to raise their arms forward during an assessment, due to the way the patient identifies with the movement.

When observing the patient's natural body movement, we want to see if the movements are smooth, or if they are unnatural and awkward. Smooth and balanced movements indicate that the patient is healthy and that the condition is likely to be mild. Movements that appear rapid and hurried indicate Heat (Re, 热) type conditions, due to the nature of Heat causing the channels to open and the Qi to become hyperactive. Patients with Heat type conditions may also appear restless and agitated, and even quite frantic. If the movements are still strong, this would indicate excess type Heat, whereas feebler movements would indicate deficiency type Heat (caused by Yin deficiency). Patients may also have a flushed complexion to the presence of Heat and the Wei Qi moving towards the surface.

Movements that appear to be slow and tense may indicate Cold (Han, 寒) type conditions due to the nature of Cold causing contraction of the Sinew channels and the inward withdrawal of the Wei Qi. As a result of the lack of circulation through the channels, due to constriction and withdrawal of the Wei Qi, stillness will occur in the channels and the patient will have reduced movement. Patients may also appear pale, or have a slight cyanotic appearance, again, due to the inward withdrawal of the Wei Qi and the constriction of the Blood vessels.

Movements that appear lethargic and sluggish may indicate Damp (Shi, 湿) type syndromes due to excess swelling within the Sinew channels and the spaces within the joints. Patients may also suffer from stiffness and tension within the joints due to the swelling causing restriction of movement. Lethargic and sluggish movements may also indicate Qi and/or Yang deficiency syndromes, due to a lack of power and activation of the limbs, although similar movements to those due to excess Damp, deficiency of Qi and/or Yang type movements will not appear as stiff or restricted, and there will be little or no swelling.

If the patient experiences uncomfortable and reduced mobility of the joints, it can indicate Qi stagnation and/or Blood stasis. If Qi stagnation and/or Blood stasis is present, the patient may also potentially be 'guarding' the area or using compensatory movements, such as a limp.

Body movement	Indication
Smooth and natural	Healthy, or the condition is mild
Rapid, hurried and restless	Heat
Slow and tense	Cold
Lethargic and sluggish, with restriction	Damp
Lethargic and sluggish, without restriction	Qi and/or Yang deficiency
Restriction with discomfort and/or pain	Qi and/or Blood stagnation

The Shen (神, Spirit) of the patient

Observation of the Shen (神) is a huge area of diagnosis, covering many aspects such as observing behaviour and body language, movement, breathing, eye diagnosis, facial diagnosis, and more. Again, there is far too much to go into detail in this book. However, the patient's general expression and demeanour will suggest the condition of their Shen, which will, in turn, give a broad indication of the disease severity. As a general rule, if the patient is in good spirits, responds sharply with good awareness, and has bright and focused eyes, then the disease is mild and has not yet affected the Shen. If, however, the patient appears spiritless, with dull eyes and is sluggish in response, then the disease is serious and it is affecting their Shen. This indicates that the condition will be difficult to treat.

Specific observations

Specific observations should be done during the consultation, and are dictated by the patient's main complaint. For example, if a patient presents with knee pain, it is important to take a look at the knee in question. Of course! This may seem obvious, however many practitioners (of various therapies) will treat without full assessment and/or diagnosis – they essentially go in blind!

When observing parts of the body, like with palpation it is important to compare the area of complaint with its healthy counterpart. For instance, we should compare the patient's injured knee to the patient's good knee. This is to assess what is perhaps 'normal' to the patient, and is useful when observing potential swellings, deformities and colouring of the tissues. The following categories are specific observations that we look for during our assessment.

Swellings or enlargements

Observation of the limbs and joints should first include looking for any swellings or enlargements, especially if trauma has occurred to the area. It is essential to identify swellings and enlargements, because it can be quite damaging to directly treat an area that is swollen if the channels flowing in and out of the area have not been opened first. It is also important that comparisons are made to the other limbs and joints, as sometimes a joint such as the ankle may look absolutely fine, until it is compared to the healthy ankle.

Swelling is actually considered to be a perfectly normal part of the healing response, and happens due to the increased flow of Wei Qi accumulating in the area, bringing along with it an increased amount of Blood and Body Fluids in order to heal the Sinew channels from injury. It is only when the body is unable to independently reabsorb the swelling, perhaps due to injury to the vessels and/or channels, that the swelling becomes an issue and help is needed. This is when swelling can become chronic, and begin to slow healing down or begin to damage the area further due to obstructing the Qi.

Atrophies or weaknesses

Tissue atrophies (meaning wasting away) or weaknesses are almost always due to a localised deficiency; however, there may be other causes that mean there is excess somewhere else along the channel, such as trauma or injury that prevents Qi and Blood flow to the atrophied muscle. To observe atrophies and weaknesses, it is important to always compare muscles and tissues to other localised muscles and tissues, and also their opposite counterparts (such as comparing the left calf to the right calf). Observing atrophies or weaknesses helps us to assess which channels are activating and functioning correctly, and which ones aren't.

Colours and/or bruising

Observing the colouration of the body tissues is important to help towards diagnosing the nature of Qi and Blood in the local area and within the corresponding channels. Colouration should be compared to the immediate surrounding tissues, in addition to the same area on the opposite side of the body.

Chapter 10 of the *Ling Shu* states that, 'blueness of the channels indicates Cold and pain (stagnation), whereas redness of the channels indicates Heat'. If the skin and body tissues have a slight cyanotic colouration, this indicates that excess Cold is present within the channel, and occurs due to the Cold causing a restriction of circulation to the area. Redness of the skin and body tissues is due to Heat or Fire causing the Qi and Blood to fill the vessels and travel to the surface. Pale skin can indicate conditions caused by a deficiency of Qi and/or Yang if white, or Blood if pale and withered. A yellow tinge in specific areas of the body can indicate an excess of Dampness within those channels. Bruising or broken vessels will indicate trauma, or Blood stasis.

Colour	Indication
Red	Heat or Fire
Pale and blue/cyanotic	Cold
Pale and white	Qi and/or Yang deficiency
Pale and withered	Blood deficiency
Yellow	Damp
Bruised	Blood stasis

Deformities and abnormalities

A deformity or abnormality is where part of the body has formed differently to how it should naturally have formed. Within the physical body, this may manifest as deformities of the bone, such as misshaped bones or bones that are sized differently, or deformities of the muscles and tissues, such as an underdeveloped muscle or misaligned muscle attachment. Some deformities or abnormalities will not cause any disruption or discomfort to the patient, have been present since birth and are perfectly harmless. However, some may cause disruption to the flow of Qi and Blood, causing pain and discomfort in addition to possible compensations of the Sinew channels in regards to movement and mobility. If the deformity or abnormality cannot be treated fully, it is often best to focus treatment at reducing any symptoms that are being caused.

Breathing patterns

Subconscious breathing patterns don't lie, and watching the patient's breathing patterns can give subtle indications to the state of balance within their body. For example, if the patient is subconsciously holding their breath slightly after inhalation and before breathing back out, it could indicate that they are Yang deficient, as this is a natural Yang tonification method. Conversely, if the patient is holding their breath momentarily after exhalation before breathing in again, it may indicate that they are Yin deficient, as this is a gentle Yin nourishing method by creating stillness within the nervous system. Sighing can indicate stagnation of Qi, and occurs as the body is subconsciously trying to release the stagnation of Qi by forcefully activating and resetting the breathing pattern of both the Lungs and Diaphragm.

In addition to the above breathing patterns, it is essential to distinguish between two other main types of breathing: diaphragmatic breathing and chest breathing (also known as apical breathing). This can be monitored when the patient is lying on their back through either observation or palpation. Diaphragmatic breathing uses the movement of the Diaphragm to engage and regulate the breath, whilst the chest barely moves at all unless the patient breathes deeply. Chest breathing, on the other hand, is a dysfunctional breathing pattern and refers to breathing that only involves the chest and upper neck, whilst the Diaphragm or abdomen is not engaged whatsoever, or at most, very little. The desired way to breathe is diaphragmatically. This is why there is such an emphasis on diaphragmatic breathing in systems such as Qi Gong, Taiji and Yoga. To breathe correctly, it is important to expand like a balloon in a 360-degree motion. This means that more muscles are involved, making it more efficient. Due to the fact that it is more efficient, respiration is slower and more relaxed.

To assess whether the patient is breathing diaphragmatically or with the chest, simply ask the patient to take a breath and observe the movement of both the chest and the abdomen. For diaphragmatic breathing, it should be the abdomen that moves first, followed by slight inflation of the chest. It is also important to observe the movement of the ribs, as they should not flare, and check that the neck muscles are not lifting the ribcage or becoming tight (both indicating chest breathing). If it is difficult to observe the patient, perhaps because they are breathing shallowly, place one of your hands on the patient's chest, with your other hand on their lower abdomen, and feel which one rises first. If the hand on the chest moves first, or if both hands move at the same time, then the patient is chest breathing.

Chest breathing only elevates the ribcage, drawing it upwards and towards the head, leading to the Diaphragm stagnating. What's more, chest breathing will generally isolate the muscles of the upper back and neck, causing them to become more Yang, leading to tension and hypertonicity. When the Diaphragm does not engage, muscles such as the sternocleidomastoid and the scalenes are utilised to help elevate the rib cage for breathing. Due to the fact that these muscles are not meant to be doing this job, the tension and hypertonicity of the upper back and neck muscles can lead to stagnation of the upper Jiao, causing headaches, neck pain and shoulder pain.

The causes of chest breathing are usually Qi stagnation from either physical or emotional trauma. If you think of someone who has lower back pain or sciatica, for instance, their breathing pattern will have altered in a way to avoid any discomfort. On the other hand, if someone has gone through emotional trauma, it is often the case that they attempt to hide or bury the emotion, which causes stagnation within the centre of the body, where the Diaphragm is located.

Key visual observations

- Posture and body movement.
- Overall Shen (神, Spirit) of the patient.
- Swellings or enlargements.
- Atrophies or weaknesses.
- Colours and/or bruising.
- Deformities or abnormalities.
- Breathing patterns.

Inquiry

During the consultation, one of the main methods of diagnosis is via inquiry – this is essentially asking the patient questions about themselves and their condition. Inquiry is one of the key methods of diagnosis, with much of the consultation spent talking with the patient about their ailment(s), history and lifestyle. However, even though it is one of the key methods of diagnosis, it is indeed one of the weakest forms of diagnosis simply due to the fact that we are relying on information given to us by the patient to be accurate and truthful. In fact, patients may omit things, forget things, or even lie in response to certain questions. It also relies on the patient understanding clearly what is being asked, and for the practitioner to be able to ask clearly and tactfully enough. This is why it is important to use inquiry as an addition to all of the other methods of diagnosis. The following pages will cover the various areas of inquiry that are relevant in regards to the assessment of the Sinew channels.

Personal information

When meeting your patient for the first time, it is important to take their personal information. This may seem like a simple formality, although actually it is helpful to the diagnosis and treatment plan. Personal information should include the patient's age (date of birth), gender and occupation. It should also include their contact information and contact details for their general practitioner (GP), although these do not help so much towards their diagnosis.

Age

The patient's age can give us a *rough* indication of potential imbalances and the strength of their constitution. It will also give us an indication of how strong we can make a treatment, and how reactive the patient is likely to be. Of course, this can only act as a rough guide, and there are many other factors that will determine a patient's condition.

Specific ages are not so important, although broader age ranges are, and it is the young and the elderly that we need to make changes to our default treatments for. Generally speaking, younger patients (aged 0–20) are likely to suffer from more excess conditions, and in particular, excess Yang type conditions. This is due to the fact that children and teenagers are in a state of 'Yang', which is necessary for the rapid growth and development that they are going through during this time. If a young patient does indeed suffer from deficiency, it is likely due to malnourishment from a poor diet, or congenital factors passed down from their parents. Younger patients are also very reactive to Tui Na or other bodywork therapies that work on the Sinew channels, due to them being in the 'Spring' stage of their lives. This is the time of life where the Qi is very active within the Sinew channel system of the body, and where the Sinew channels are developing and strengthening, and therefore easily repaired. For this reason, it is not necessary to give strong treatments to younger patients, and the number of treatments needed is likely to be fewer.

Elderly patients (considered to be aged 60 onwards) are more likely to suffer from deficiency type conditions, and are more likely to be constitutionally weaker in general. This means that treatment should be softer and more gentle. Older patients will also likely need more sessions as they may be less reactive to treatment. This is simply because many diseases or causes of disease in elderly patients are longstanding and due to an underlying condition that has been present for many years. Generally speaking, the longer a patient has harboured a condition, the longer it will take to treat.

Gender

As with the patient's age, the gender of the patient will give us a general idea of what imbalances are *potentially* present. This still doesn't mean that certain imbalances *will* be present.

Women tend to suffer from deficiency more readily than men. This is largely due to the three bodily processes of menstruation, gestation and lactation. During all three processes, women draw on a lot of Blood. This also places strain on the Spleen Qi and both Kidney Qi and Jing (精). Over the years of monthly menstruation, and the possibility of conceiving and having children, the Vital Substances of a woman are likely to become deficient unless much focus has been put on health preservation and leading a healthy lifestyle.

Men, on the other hand, are more likely to suffer from excess type conditions and stagnation. This is due to the fact that men are said to be 'governed by Qi', and also that they are more Yang in nature. This, again, is just generalising, and should not be taken as fact for every patient.

Occupation

The occupation of the patient is an important piece of information to find out, as it will tell us a great deal about the kinds of conditions the patient spends much of their time being exposed to. It will also tell us how much or how little activity they are doing day to day, in addition to what type of activity it is. Some patients' occupations may cause them to develop poor posture, such as office work or occupations that entail working in tight spaces. Consistently positioned in a certain posture with lack of movement will cause tightening of the Sinew channels, and often cause stagnation at certain parts of the body. For example, excessive sitting in a chair may cause stagnation of the Liver Qi (due to lack of movement), stagnation of the Intestines (due to being bent at the waist), and deficiency of the Stomach and Bladder Sinew channels (due to inactivity and disengagement). If using a computer, the same position may additionally create tension along the Small Intestine Sinew channel due to elevation of the arms, creating discomfort in the neck and shoulder. This shows just how dangerous an office job can be!

In addition to a 'lack of' movement, excessive movement can also take its toll. Occupations that entail repeated movements may cause stagnation and overstrain of the Sinew channels, resulting in repetitive strain conditions or excessive tension as well as various deficiencies. For example, repeatedly lifting heavy objects may damage the lower back by injuring the Bladder Sinew channel in addition to weakening the Kidney Qi.

Other occupations may also expose the patient to certain climatic factors from the environment – an example of this would be farming, where the patient may be exposed to excessive Cold, Damp or Heat depending on the climate of their location. Climatic factors don't only refer to the physical weather, but also the working environment. For example, in Classical Chinese Medicine, a stressful environment would also be classed as a climatic factor, corresponding to Wind. Working in a stressful environment would create tension within the Sinew channels by causing them to contract slightly in attempt to 'protect' the patient. Over time, this will cause tension and stiffness to certain Sinew channels, often manifesting as pain and discomfort.

Main complaint and the onset of symptoms

As obvious as it may sound, one of the main areas of inquiry is to question the patient about their main complaint, which is the reason that they have come to see you for treatment. This includes any signs and symptoms that are directly associated with the patient's main complaint, such as types of pain, as described at the beginning of this section, in addition to asking if anything in particular makes the condition better or worse.

In regards to dysfunction of the Sinew channels, it is also necessary to ask the patient about the 'perceived' location of their main complaint, as this helps to identify which channel(s) is involved (I say 'perceived', as where the patient *thinks* the problem is, isn't always correct). It should also be asked if there are any radiating sensations (pain, numbness, tingling, etc.), or any limitations in movement, as this can also help to identify which Sinew channels are involved.

Asking the patient about the main complaint should also include asking about the onset of symptoms. Questioning about the onset of symptoms would involve asking when the symptoms occurred (assessing the condition as being acute or chronic), what happened to cause the symptoms (in the case of an injury or accident, asking about the way the body moved during the incident), and if the symptoms came about gradually (indicating a deficient or Yin condition) or suddenly (indicating an excess or Yang condition).

The Ten Questions

Within Chinese Medicine, inquiry also involves going through what are known as the 'Ten Questions'. These are not so much a list of questions, but ten areas of questioning (which could end up as hundreds of questions!). The Ten Questions are:

- hot or cold/chills and fever

- sweating

- sleep

- pain

- emotions

- head and face (including the senses)

- chest, abdomen and limbs

- appetite, thirst and taste (including diet)

- bowels and urination

- menstruation (including male sexual health).

These allow us to delve deeper into what is happening with our patients, and encourage them to tell us things that they would not necessarily think would be relevant. I am not going to go into each of the Ten Questions here, as this would be more suited to a book that specifically focuses on Chinese Medicine diagnostics only – it is a topic large enough to fill a whole book in its own right. Information on the Ten Questions can be found in any reputable book on Chinese Medicine diagnostics.

Medical history

In addition to the Ten Questions and inquiry about the complaint, it is important to ask about the patient's medical history, including any past illnesses or medical interventions (such as surgeries), in addition to any family-related illnesses that may have been passed down from either parent. It is also important here to take note of any medications that the patient is taking, as many have a detrimental effect on the body when taken for long periods of time. For example, commonly prescribed antibiotics are known to damage the Spleen's ability to transform Dampness, leaving the patient prone to Damp in the channels, whereas statins (another commonly prescribed drug) are thought to damage the Spleen and Liver, causing stagnation and Heat.

Areas of inquiry

- Personal information.

- Main complaint.

- Onset of the complaint (including a description of how it happened).

- The Ten Questions.

- Medical history (to include past and present medications).

Palpation

Palpation is the method of using the hands to examine and assess the body through touch. Alongside observational diagnosis, it is considered to be one of the strongest and most reliable methods of diagnosis, with the most accurate and comprehensive aspect of palpation being Chinese Medicine pulse diagnosis.

When palpating the body, we are essentially palpating the body tissues and the Sinew channels on a physical level, which reflect the state of Qi and Blood on an energetic level. There are indeed ways to palpate the energetic body without physical touch, although this is a whole subject in its own right. With palpation, it is important that we always palpate both the diseased areas of the body and the healthy areas. This is so that we can make comparisons, such as in temperature or tonicity, in order to help strengthen our diagnosis.

Palpating the channels for temperature and tonicity

When assessing the Sinew channels with palpation, we will immediately be able to notice the temperature of the skin, and also the tonicity of the skin and muscles. This is a reflection of the Qi and Blood within the channels. When feeling the temperature and tonicity of the channels, it is important to compare against other parts of the body to ensure that it is indeed a channel-related issue rather than their overall constitution.

The feeling of warmth indicates that Heat is present, whereas the feeling of coldness or lack of warmth (there should be slight warmth to the skin) will indicate that Cold is present in the channels, or that there is stagnation somewhere along the channel, preventing Qi and Blood flow to the area.

When palpating the tonicity of the channels, we are looking for either hypertonicity (indicating an excess) or hypotonicity (indicating a deficiency). Often if there is hypertonicity of one channel, there will be hypotonicity of another channel, such is the nature of Yin and Yang. This may cause an imbalance of movement and support, thus causing further injury to the channels due to compensation and adjustment. Hypertonicity can lead to stagnation, as it creates difficulty for the Qi and Blood to flow in and out of the tissues, therefore creating the feeling of pain or discomfort due to excess (Shi, 实) type that would be made worse by applying pressure. Hypotonicity, on the other hand, can also lead to stagnation, as the Qi and Blood circulation is not ample to flow freely or strongly enough. This also leads to the feeling of pain or discomfort, this time of deficient (Xu, 虚) type, and would be alleviated by pressure. If the channels feel flaccid and 'squashy', this may indicate Dampness or Phlegm within the channels. Phlegm will also manifest as lumps and nodules under the skin. Dampness and Phlegm may also cause numbness along the channel(s) due to the obstruction of Qi and Blood.

Palpation of specific points

There are certain points on the body, for various reasons, that are useful for narrowing down a diagnosis and giving us insight into which channels or organs are suffering from disease. The main points used for diagnosis by palpation are the Front Mu (募) points, the Back Shu (輸) points, and Ashi (啊是) points, as these often become sore when their related channel or organ is out of balance.

Palpation of the Front Mu (募) and Back Shu (輸) points

Classically speaking, palpation of the Front Mu points is often used as a diagnostic tool for acute conditions of the *channels* (however, they are also thought to communicate directly to their corresponding organ), whereas the Back Shu points are more often palpated as a diagnostic tool for chronic conditions of the *organs*. Classically, it was said that the Mu points were used for 'Yang' diseases (meaning acute and external), whereas the Shu points were used for 'Yin' diseases (meaning chronic and internal). Upon palpation, if there is an imbalance with one or more of the channels and/or organs, the corresponding Front Mu point(s) or Back Shu point(s) will often illicit a sensitive reaction, such as pain or tenderness. Techniques such as An Fa or Rou Fa may also be used on these points to help regulate the corresponding channels and/or organs. For example, stimulation of LU-1 (Zhong Fu) and BL-13 (Fei Shu) can help to open the chest and relieve tightness of breath.

Mu (募) means to gather, and is where the Qi of the corresponding channel gathers and emerges. The Mu points are sometimes referred to as 'alarm' points due to the fact they become sensitive during times of disease, and were classically said to treat

'Yang' diseases, meaning acute and external diseases (external relating to the channels and collaterals).

Shu (輸) means to transport or to deliver, and Shu points are thought to deliver Yang Qi directly from the Du channel to the corresponding organ. They are classically said to treat 'Yin' diseases, meaning chronic and internal diseases (internal relating to the organs), and do so by tonifying and regulating the corresponding organ to bring it back to balance.

A list of the Front Mu and Back Shu points can be found below:

Organ	Front Mu (募) point	Back Shu (輸) point*
Lung	LU-1	BL-13
Pericardium	R-17	BL-14
Heart	R-14	BL-15
Diaphragm	–	BL-17
Liver	Lv-14	BL-18
Gall Bladder	GB-24	BL-19
Spleen	Lv-13	BL-20
Stomach	R-12	BL-21
San Jiao	R-5	BL-22
Kidney	GB-25	BL-23
Large Intestine	ST-25	BL-25
Small Intestine	R-4	BL-27
Bladder	R-3	BL-28

* Note: Not all Back Shu (輸) points have been listed here.

Palpation of Ashi (啊是) points

When palpating the Sinew channels themselves, we are first looking for what are called Ashi (啊是) points (pronounced Ah-Sherr). These are points that may occur anywhere on the body that feel sensitive, tender or painful to the patient once palpated or pressed. Ashi points may also feel flaccid/weak, tight/stuck, cold/hot in the immediate area to the practitioner. The literal meaning of Ashi is 'Ah yes!', and is so called due to the patient feeling discomfort when the point or area is palpated or pressed, and wanting to let the practitioner know. They may or may not be located on specific channels or at specific acupoints. Essentially they can appear anywhere on the body, and indicate the possible root of disease and the area where treatment should be carried out.

Ashi points are most commonly located close to the surface of the body, which can be felt easily by palpation, and is a key method of diagnosis. However, some Ashi points may occur on a deeper level, such as within a joint where it is impossible to palpate, although the patient can feel it themselves. Asking the patient about the nature of the sensation can also help to diagnose. Once an Ashi point has been located, it is important that the channel that it is located along is identified in order to treat the Sinew channel successfully. Occasionally, an Ashi point may lie in an area where two or more Sinew channels overlap, in which case treatment should be given to all Sinew channels involved.

Ashi (啊是) point sensations

- Sudden increased pain on palpation.

- Flaccid or weak tissue.*

- Tightness within the tissues.*

- Feeling of cold on palpation.*

- Feeling of heat on palpation.*

* These sensations are only felt within the immediate area.

Chapter 6

Assessment of the Sinew Channels through Movement and Engagement

Each classical pairing of the Sinew channels (discussed in Section 1) enables us to move in certain ways. If one or more of the channels is injured or suffering from disease (such as from external pathogenic factors), there may be restricted, uncomfortable, or even painful movement. When assessing each patient, it is important to go through what are known as the 'basic movements' of each specific channel and observe how the patient is able to move. More detailed ailments of each Sinew channel can be found within Chapter 13 of the *Ling Shu*, and are discussed in Section 1 of this book, although the following discusses the general movement of each Sinew channel.

Pairing of the Sinew channels

Tai Yang (Bladder and Small Intestine) Sinew channels

The Tai Yang channels are located on the posterior aspect of the body and are mainly related to our upright posture and the movement of extension. It is the Tai Yang channels that enable us to extend outwards whilst also acting as our first line of defence. (If you think of when we shield ourselves from something being thrown at us, for instance, it is often with our Tai Yang channels that we do so.)

The leg aspect of the Tai Yang Sinew channel (Bladder) is what gives us a strong posture and the ability to stand tall with our head held high, which is also why it is linked closely with our self-esteem and self-confidence.

The arm aspect of the Tai Yang Sinew channel (Small Intestine), on the other hand, enables us to lift the arms up and extend them outwards in front (with extension travelling through the little finger), as if reaching out for something. Another common action of this channel is to hold the arms up and forwards in order to hold on to a steering wheel or to type at a computer. It is also the Small Intestine Sinew channel that gives us correct engagement of the scapula to stabilise the entire shoulder joint through the rotator cuff.

When the Tai Yang channels are injured, there may be pain that occurs on extension, stiffness or discomfort that occurs when the patient stands upright from a seated position or an inability to stand tall. This pain will be experienced during movement, whereas resting will relieve symptoms. In regards to pathogenic factors, the Tai Yang channels are first to be affected during external invasions such as the common cold or the flu.

Shao Yang (Gall Bladder and San Jiao) Sinew channels

The Shao Yang channels are located to the sides of the body, and are related to our ability to rotate. This includes free rotation of the torso, rotation of the limbs and rotation and side bending of the neck/head.

The movement of the leg aspect of the Shao Yang Sinew channel (Gall Bladder) helps to keep the body in alignment in regards to rotation of the hips and the legs, and balancing the Yin and Yang relationship of the body. This can clearly be seen when we rotate our body at the waist, and also when turning our legs and feet inwards or outwards from the hip. The Gall Bladder Sinew channel also activates lateral abduction of the legs.

Movement of the arm aspect of the Shao Yang Sinew channel (San Jiao), on the other hand, can be clearly seen in rotation of the arms on a central axis (in a pronating/supinating manner such as using a screwdriver or turning a door handle), lateral abduction of the arm and turning or tilting the head to one side. It also assists in the movement of the opening and closing of the jaw and movement of the tempo-mandibular joint due to the channel trajectory passing over the lower jaw and in front of the ears.

When the Shao Yang channels are injured or not working correctly, the patient may not have correct rotational movement, or the limbs will be either under- or over-rotated. For example, when the Leg Shao Yang (Gall Bladder) channel is in a state of hyper- or hypotonicity, the leg may be rotated slightly outwards or inwards respectively. Equally, if the Shao Yang channels are affecting the upper part of the body such as the arms, head and neck, then the patient may not be able to laterally abduct the arm, supinate/pronate the arm or rotate or laterally tilt the head without discomfort.

Yang Ming (Stomach and Large Intestine) Sinew channels

The Yang Ming channels are located on the anterior aspect of the body, and are mainly related to our ability to brace ourselves and to bear weight, in addition to reaching out. They maintain a Yin/Yang (front/back) relationship with the Tai Yang channels in assisting the Tai Yang channels to keep our posture strong. They essentially work in the same way that we understand our core works to maintain a stable posture.

The movement of the leg aspect of the Yang Ming Sinew channel (Stomach) can be clearly seen when a baby is learning to crawl, with the legs used to push away and propel the body forwards whilst bracing the core. (It is said within Chinese Medicine that a child will develop their ability to stand strong through the act of crawling.) The Stomach channel also maintains a Yin/Yang (front/back) relationship with the Bladder Sinew channels in assisting the Bladder Sinew channel to keep our posture strong and upright, especially when standing still. They essentially work together in the same way that we understand our core works with our back to maintain a stable posture. The arm aspect of the Yang Ming Sinew channel (Large Intestine), on the other hand, is unique among the Sinew channels in that it has both a Yin and Yang movement. It is the Large Intestine Sinew channel that gives the ability to lift the arms in front in order to push away, but also to bring objects towards us. It is essentially the Large Intestine Sinew channel that acts as the interaction between the outward movement of Yang and the pulling inward movement of Yin (which is why the Large Intestine Sinew channel is the final Yang Sinew channel before the Wei Qi (衛氣) circulates through the Yin Sinew channels).

When the Yang Ming channels are not working as they should, the patient may not be able to stand still without discomfort or pain. The patient will be forced to collapse at the waist when standing still, and will not be able to hold any weight out in front of them. The patient should, however, feel okay to stand up straight when walking forward due to the Tai Yang channels taking over. This is a key differentiation to help in diagnosing back pain due to either the Tai Yang channels or the Yang Ming channels.

Tai Yin (Spleen and Lung) Sinew channels

The Tai Yin channels are the first of the Yin channels, and are located on the medial aspects of the limbs and the torso. They are involved in the inward movement of the limbs towards the body.

Movement of the leg aspect of the Tai Yin Sinew channels (Spleen) involves bringing the lower limbs inwards towards the body, and can be seen as we go to sit down by bending at the waist and lowering ourselves steadily into a chair, or by lifting our knees up to our torso. It is the Spleen Sinew channel that also gives structure and support to the arches of the feet and stability to the medial aspect of the ankle.

The arm aspect of the Tai Yin Sinew channels (Lung), on the other hand, involves bringing the arm inwards towards the body, and can be seen when carrying something out in front with the palms facing upwards (as if carrying a pizza). Strength in the Lung Sinew channel also helps to support good posture and alignment of the shoulders, and keeps the chest open by preventing a collapse of the shoulders and chest. The Lung Sinew channel is also important for the breath. This is not only because the channel helps to open up the chest, as mentioned above, but also due to the fact that the channel acts on and engages both the intercostals and the Diaphragm.

When the Tai Yin channels have been affected by injury or the invasion of pathogens, the patient will find it difficult to make movements towards the centre of the body, such as bringing the knees up to the abdomen or chest. An example of this would be when a patient is unable to smoothly transition from a standing position to a seated position without discomfort or collapsing into a chair. Less commonly, the patient will also find it uncomfortable to bring the arms inwards towards the body, experiencing discomfort in the arms or the chest muscles.

Shao Yin (Kidney and Heart) Sinew channels

In regards to functional movement, whereas the Shao Yang Sinew channels act as the *external* pivot (therefore lateral rotation), the Shao Yin Sinew channels are sometimes considered to act as the *internal* pivot, and therefore govern medial rotation. The Shao Yin Sinew channels also assist the Shao Yang Sinew channels in rotation of the torso, and do so from within the core of the body (notice that the Kidney Sinew channel travels deep within the body and ascends upwards within the spine).

The movement of the leg aspect of the Shao Yin Sinew channel (Kidney) can be clearly seen during inward rotation of the hips, in a movement that in the Chinese Arts is called 'closing the Kua' (the Kua in this context refers roughly to the region around the internal hip joint and the inguinal crease). In certain Chinese Arts, such as Qi Gong and Taiji, the movement of 'closing the Kua' involves activation and engagement of the Kidney Sinew channels. When the Kidney Sinew channels are engaged too much, for instance, in a pigeon-toed stance, this causes tension in the lumbar aspect of the Kidney Sinew channel and is actually thought to close the fascia around the Ming Men.

The movement of the arm aspect of the Shao Yin Sinew channel (Heart) governs internal rotation of the arms. In regards to the upper limbs, the Heart Sinew channel governs the complex movement of rotation and flexion. This movement can be seen, for example, when pouring a kettle of water, or bringing a cup towards the mouth and drinking. The Heart Sinew channel also has an internal connection up towards the root of the tongue and connects with the corners of the mouth, allowing free movement of the tongue and the ability to smile. It is said that smiling engages the tissues around the Heart and opens up the spaces around it.

When the Shao Yin channels are injured there will be pain or discomfort with the complex movement of rotation combined with flexion of a joint. For example, when there is injury to the Arm Shao Yin (Heart) sinew channel, there will be pain at the elbow that is made worse by flexion and rotation (this may present as golfer's elbow – medial epicondylitis).

Jue Yin (Liver and Pericardium) Sinew channels

Some consider the Jue Yin Sinew channels to be the inner most aspect of the body, and the deepest of the channel pairings. It is important to note that within Chinese Medicine, the term 'deepest' does not necessarily mean depth as in physical location, but in the way that the body functions. The Jue Yin Sinew channels are responsible for the movement of adduction, in addition to giving the ability to hold and support the body whilst relaxing in a lying-down position. The Jue Yin Sinew channels are also in control of the finer motor movements, which is why there can be a tremor or incoordination when the Jue Yin channels become dysfunctional, and also why the Jue Yin Sinew channels are considered to be the 'deepest' Sinew channels. As the deepest channel pairing, the Jue Yin Sinew channels are also responsible for the internal connective tissues that emerge from the area around the Gao Huang region, and engage the core to give it stability. This, in turn, helps the circulation of the Vital Substances within the body and helps to guide them to and through the extremities. This is reflected in the Liver and Pericardium functions of assisting in the circulation of the Vital Substances from the centre of the body.

The leg aspect of the Jue Yin Sinew (Liver) channel is specifically responsible for adduction of the hip in addition to assisting in laterally rotating and flexing the thigh. It also engages with the lower abdomen and assists with contraction of the genitals to help with both arousal and prevention of flaccidity. The Liver Sinew channel is also responsible for the finer motor movements between the torso and the lower limbs, therefore giving the ability to make smooth and coordinated movements. This is reflected in the Liver's function of maintaining the smooth flow of Qi.

The arm aspect of the Jue Yin Sinew (Pericardium) channel is specifically responsible for adduction of the upper limbs, in addition to clenching a fist and helping to support the Diaphragm. Similar to the Liver Sinew channel in regard to the lower limbs and trunk, it is also responsible for the finer motor movements of the upper limbs and trunk. This gives the ability to make smooth and coordinated movements, including with our breathing. What's more, the Pericardium Sinew channel also has a key responsibility for the internal connective tissues that open the chest, which in turn helps the circulation of the Vital Substances within the body and helps to guide them to and through the extremities.

The main sign of dysfunction of the Jue Yin Sinew channels as a pairing is tremor or uncoordinated movements, in addition to a weakness or inability to perform adduction movements. Classically, it was also said that there would be paralysis when the Jue Yin Sinew channels were injured. This is thought to be due to the connection of the Jue Yin Sinew channels to the Gao Huang region at the centre of the body.

Assessment of the Sinew channels through strength and engagement

In addition to observing the patient's movements as described above, it is important to check the strength and engagement of suspected dysfunctional channels. This is essentially a reflection of the transmission of Qi through the channel. If there is weakness or discomfort of a channel during active engagement, it demonstrates an obstruction and stagnation within the channel. Strength and engagement assessments clearly demonstrate to both the practitioner and the patient that there is something wrong. It is a good way to get a clear idea of where an injury may be, as pain is not always a clear indicator of an injury location. Some Sinew channels have multiple assessments due to the length of each channel and the various regions that they pass and bind to.

When performing strength and engagement assessments to the Sinew channels, it is important to be mindful that if there is an issue with a Yin channel, it is often compensated by a Yang channel (and vice versa) or a channel on the opposite side of the body. What's more, if the patient experiences any pain or stagnation when doing these assessments, stop, as there is no need to go any further. There is a wide range of strength and engagement assessments for the Sinew channels, although below are a number of basic yet key assessments for each of the Sinew channels.

Leg Tai Yang (Bladder) Sinew channel

Due to the fact that the Bladder Sinew channel is so long, spanning the entire posterior of the body, it has more assessments than the other channels. To test the strength and transmission of Qi through the Bladder Sinew channels, perform the following assessments:

Assessment One

The first assessment of the Bladder Sinew channel is to check the patient's ability to extend the spine, focusing on the lumbar area. Ask the patient to lie face up in a relaxed supine position, with their knees locked straight. Take hold of the patient's heel, and slowly lift the heels up, 7–15 cm. Ask the patient to push their heels down into your hands whilst you resist. This will engage the patient's Bladder Sinew channel. The patient should be able to hold a straight plank position. If there is pain or weakness, this may indicate a dysfunction somewhere in the Bladder Sinew channel.

Assessment Two

The second assessment is to check the patient's neck extension. Ask the patient to lie face down in a relaxed prone position, and place your hand on the back of the patient's head at the occiput. Ask the patient to extend the neck by pushing their head back into your hand whilst you resist. The patient should be able to hold this position comfortably without pain or any shaking. Pain, discomfort, weakness or shaking indicates a dysfunction of the Bladder Sinew channel.

Assessment Three

The third assessment is to check the patient's glute muscles, as these are the strongest and largest muscles of the Bladder Sinew channel. Ask the patient to lie in a relaxed supine position, with one leg flexed, knee bent and foot flat on the bed; the other leg can be relaxed and straight. Slightly rotate the foot externally to cause rotation of the tibia and engage the glutes. Place your hand under the patient's foot, and ask the patient to drive their foot down into the bed whilst you gently lift to create some counter tension. The patient should be strong enough to be able to keep their foot in contact with the bed. Pain, discomfort or weakness indicates a dysfunction of the Bladder Sinew channel.

Assessment Four

The fourth and last assessment focuses on the mid back and lower part of the trapezius muscle. Ask the patient to lie face down in a prone position with one arm held above their head at around 45 degrees, with the elbow locked (as if they are creating a 'Y' shape with one arm). Place your hand on top of the patient's forearm, and ask the patient to push their arm backwards towards the ceiling whilst you gently resist. Again, pain, discomfort or weakness will indicate a weakness of the Bladder Sinew channel.

Arm Tai Yang (Small Intestine) Sinew Channel

The Small Intestine Sinew channels support the movement of the arms through the scapula. To assess the strength and transmission of Qi through the Small Intestine Sinew channels, perform the following assessments:

Assessment One

The first assessment of the Small Intestine Sinew channel aims to check the subscapularis muscle of the scapula. With the patient in a seated position, ask them to keep their elbow by their side whilst they hold their forearm out at 90 degrees. Place one hand on the patient's elbow to secure it in place, and the other hand on the inside of their wrist. Ask the patient to internally rotate their arm to engage the subscapularis whilst you resist. Weakness, discomfort or pain may indicate a dysfunction of the Small Intestine Sinew channel.

Assessment Two

The second assessment helps to check the arm aspect of the channel (passing through the triceps muscle) in addition to the scapula region (passing through the anterior deltoid and the trapezius muscles). Ask the patient to lie in a relaxed supine position with their arms by their waist – the palms must be face up and relaxed, to slightly stretch the channel. Take hold of the back of the patient's wrist and lift their arm towards the ceiling whilst the patient resists and attempts to keep their arm straight. The patient should be able to comfortably hold their arm in place. Weakness, pain or discomfort may indicate a dysfunction within the Small Intestine channel.

Assessment Three

The third assessment checks the strength of the upper and middle back aspect of the channel and the ability to 'spread' the arms. Ask the patient to assume a seated position with their hands interlocked behind their neck, and elbows together in front of them, about one fist apart. With both hands, gently hold the outside of the patient's elbows, and ask them to separate their elbows outwards whilst you resist. Weakness, discomfort or pain will indicate that there is a dysfunction within the Small Intestine Sinew channel.

Leg Shao Yang (Gall Bladder) Sinew Channel

The Gall Bladder Sinew channels govern external rotation of the torso and the legs, in addition to lateral abduction of the legs. To test the strength and transmission of Qi through the Gall Bladder Sinew channels, perform the following assessments:

Assessment One

The first assessment of the Gall Bladder Sinew channel is to check the external rotation of the torso. Ask the patient to straddle the bed, with one leg hanging down each side of the bed to stabilise their hips. (If this is not possible, ask the patient to sit in a reverse position on a chair.) From behind, take hold of the patient's left shoulder with your left hand, and place your right hand behind their right shoulder. This is to stop the patient from rotating to the right. Ask the patient to rotate their torso to the right whilst you resist. Weakness or pain in the intercostal or hip regions may indicate a dysfunction in the Gall Bladder Sinew channel and its ability to externally rotate. Repeat this on both sides.

Assessment Two

The second assessment is to check the ability to externally rotate the lower limbs. Ask the patient to lie face up in a relaxed supine position, with their knees bent at around 90 degrees and their feet flat on the bed. With the knees roughly one fist width apart, gently hold the lateral aspects of the knees and ask the patient to separate their knees whilst you resist. Pain, discomfort or weakness indicates a dysfunction in the Gall Bladder Sinew channel.

Assessment Three

The third assessment is to check the strength of lateral abduction in the legs. Again, ask your patient to lie face up in a supine position with one leg slightly abducted at around 30 degrees. Rotate the patient's foot inward slightly to tighten the Gall Bladder Sinew channel and put your hand on the lateral side of the ankle. Ask the patient to abduct their leg whilst you resist. Pain, discomfort or weakness indicates a dysfunction in the Gall Bladder Sinew channel.

Arm Shao Yang (San Jiao) Sinew Channel

The San Jiao Sinew channels govern our ability to rotate our arms on a central axis (in a pronating/supinating manner), laterally abduct the arms, and to rotate the head from side to side. To test the strength and transmission of Qi through the San Jiao Sinew channels, perform the following assessments:

Assessment One

The first assessment of the San Jiao Sinew channel is to check the rotation of the neck. Ask the patient to lie down in a relaxed supine position, and rotate their head to the left (this will be to assess the *right* San Jiao Sinew channel). Lift the patient's head slightly with your left hand, and place your right hand on the right side of the patient's forehead. Ask the patient to lift their head upwards against your hand whilst you apply light pressure. Pain, discomfort or weakness indicates a dysfunction in the San Jiao Sinew channel. Repeat this on the other side to check the *left* San Jiao Sinew channel.

Assessment Two

The second assessment is to check the lateral abduction of the arm. Ask your patient to take a standing or seated position, with their arm laterally abducted at around

30 degrees from their body. Place your hand on the lateral aspect of the patient's wrist, and apply light pressure. Ask the patient to push against your hand in a lateral plane whilst you resist. Pain, discomfort or weakness will indicate a dysfunction in the San Jiao Sinew channel.

Leg Yang Ming (Stomach) Sinew channel

The Stomach Sinew channels govern our ability to maintain a stable posture by bracing ourselves in addition to pushing off with our legs. To test the strength and transmission of Qi through the Stomach Sinew channels, perform the following assessments:

Assessment One

The first assessment of the Stomach Sinew channel checks the ability to flex the neck and to support the head in a neutral position. Ask the patient to lie down face up in a relaxed supine position. Bring the patient's head up into flexion, roughly 7 cm from the bed, and support their head by holding the occiput with your left hand. With your other hand, apply light pressure to the top of the patient's forehead and ask the patient to resist and further flex their neck. Pain, discomfort or weakness indicates a dysfunction in the Stomach Sinew channel.

Assessment Two

The second assessment assesses the ability for the patient to brace their anterior and their core in order to support the back. Ask the patient to lie face up in a relaxed supine position and to lift their left foot around 15 cm off the bed with their leg locked straight. Apply gentle pressure to the top of their ankle, and ask the patient to lift their foot further against your hand whilst you resist. Pain, discomfort or weakness indicates a dysfunction in the Stomach Sinew channel. Repeat this on the right side.

Assessment Three

The third assessment checks the lower leg aspect of the Stomach Sinew channel. With the patient lying face up in a relaxed supine position, place both hands around the patient's foot and pull down, placing the foot into extension. Ask the patient to dorsi flex the foot against your counter pressure. Pain, discomfort or weakness indicates a dysfunction in the Stomach Sinew channel. Repeat this on the other foot.

Arm Yang Ming (Large Intestine) Sinew channel

The Large Intestine Sinew channel is unique among the Sinew channels in a way that it has both a Yin and Yang movement. It is the Large Intestine Sinew channel that gives the ability to lift the arms in front in order to push away, but also to bring objects towards us. To test the strength and transmission of Qi through the Large Intestine Sinew channels, perform the following assessments:

Assessment One

The first assessment for the Large Intestine Sinew channel is to check the anterior raise of the arm and strength of the shoulder aspect of the channel. Ask the patient to lie face up in a relaxed supine position with their arm raised in front of them at around 30–45 degrees. Place your hand on top of the patient's hand, and add gentle pressure whilst the patient resists. Ask the patient to push up against your hand whilst you apply counter pressure. Weakness or pain indicates a dysfunction with the Large Intestine Sinew channel.

Note: The patient's hand and wrist are kept relaxed during Assessment One, and the patient should *not* form a fist.

Assessment Two

The second assessment is to check the flexion of the elbow. In a standing position, ask the patient to place their elbow by their side and hold their forearm out at 90 degrees with their palm facing inwards and their thumb tucked in (this slightly disengages the Lung Sinew channel and prioritises the Large Intestine Sinew channel). Place your hand on top of their wrist, and ask the patient to lift their hand towards their bicep whilst keeping their elbow tucked in (like a bicep curl) whilst you resist. Weakness or pain indicates a dysfunction with the Large Intestine Sinew channel.

Note: It is important that during Assessment Two the patient has their palm facing inwards (rather than upwards) with the thumb tucked in, otherwise the Lung Sinew channel will be engaged rather than the Large Intestine Sinew channel.

Leg Tai Yin (Spleen) Sinew channel

The Spleen Sinew channels hold up the arches of the feet in addition to bringing the legs up and into the torso, and supporting the core tissues. To test the strength and transmission of Qi through the Spleen Sinew channels, perform the following assessments:

Assessment One

The first assessment of the Spleen Sinew channel checks the strength and engagement of the patient's core. Ask the patient to lie face up in a supine position, with their knees up and feet flat on the bed. Place your arm across the patient's knees to help them stabilise, and ask the patient to bring their torso up towards the knees, as if doing a sit-up. Place your other arm across the patient's chest and apply gentle downward pressure whilst the patient resists. The patient should be able to comfortably hold their position. Weakness or pain indicates a dysfunction with the Spleen Sinew channel.

Assessment Two

The second assessment checks the patient's strength and ability in bringing their lower limbs inwards toward the torso. Ask the patient to take a standing position with their feet touching together whilst resting their hand on your shoulder for stability. Next, ask the patient to bring their leg into flexion by raising the knee to around hip height. Place your hand on the patient's knee and apply gentle downward pressure whilst the patient resists. The patient should be able to comfortably hold their position. Weakness or pain indicates a dysfunction with the Spleen Sinew channel. Another key sign to observe here is any vulnerability or difficulty lifting the leg into flexion to hip height.

Arm Tai Yin (Lung) Sinew channel

The Lung Sinew channels support the posture of the shoulders in addition to engaging the Diaphragm and the inward movement of the arm towards the chest. To assess the strength and transmission of Qi through the Lung Sinew channels, perform the following assessments:

Assessment One

The first assessment for the Lung Sinew channel is to check the patient's breathing and engagement of the diaphragm. Ask the patient to lie in a relaxed supine position, and place one hand on the chest and the other on their abdomen. Allow the patient to breathe in a relaxed manner with their eyes closed. Observe which hand moves first. The hand on the abdomen should rise first, before the hand on the chest. This is the correct form of breathing known as diaphragmatic breathing (as mentioned earlier). The incorrect way of breathing, which is called chest breathing (or apical breathing), is where the hand on the chest elevates first. This indicates a dysfunction with the Lung Sinew channels.

Assessment Two

The second assessment is to check the inward contraction of the arm. In a standing position, ask the patient to place their elbow by their side and hold their forearm out at 90 degrees with their palm facing upward. Place your hand onto their palm, and ask the patient to lift their palm whilst keeping their elbow tucked in (like a bicep curl) whilst you resist. Weakness or pain indicates a dysfunction with the Lung Sinew channel.

Note: It is important that during Assessment Two the patient has their palm facing upwards rather than inwards, otherwise the Large Intestine Sinew channel will be engaged rather than the Lung Sinew channel.

Leg Shao Yin (Kidney) Sinew channel

The Kidney Sinew channel is unique in that it enters deep into the body and ascends up the entire spine into the occiput. To assess the strength and transmission of Qi through the Kidney Sinew channels, perform the following assessments:

Assessment One

The first assessment of the Kidney Sinew channel is to check the internal rotation of the torso due to the aspect of Sinew channel that attaches to the Spine. Ask the patient to straddle the bed, with one leg hanging down each side of the bed to stabilise their hips.

(If this is not possible, ask the patient to sit in a reverse position on a chair.) Ask the patient to rotate their torso to the left whilst placing their right hand on their left knee. Place your hand on their left shoulder, and ask them to rotate back to a neutral position whilst you resist. Weakness or pain in the spine may indicate a dysfunction in the Kidney Sinew channel and its ability to internally rotate.

Note: Due to the fact that the Kidney Sinew channel ascends the entire Spine, any abnormal curvatures of the Spine (discussed later in 'Special examinations', Chapter 7) may be attributed to tightness within the Kidney Sinew channel. Headaches may also be a sign of tightness within the Kidney Sinew channel for this same reason.

Assessment Two
The second assessment is to test the internal rotation of the leg and the ability to close the Kua (roughly referring to the area around the hip joint and the inguinal crease). Ask the patient to sit in a relaxed supine position with one leg straight, and the other leg bent slightly and externally rotated to around 45 degrees. Place your hand on the medial aspect of the patient's bent knee and ask your patient to rotate the leg at the hip back to a neutral position whilst you resist. If there is weakness, discomfort or pain, it may indicate that the Kidney Sinew channel is dysfunctional.

Arm Shao Yin (Heart) Sinew channel
The Heart Sinew channel controls the complex movement of bringing the arms in at the same time as rotating them (place the palm of your hand in the centre of your chest, to feel your heart; this movement requires engagement of the Heart Sinews). Key strength and engagement assessments of the Heart Sinew channel would be:

Assessment One
As with the Lung Sinew channel, the first assessment for the Heart Sinew channel should be to check the patient's breathing pattern and engagement of the diaphragm. Ask the patient to lie in a relaxed supine position, and place one hand on the chest and the other on their abdomen. Allow the patient to breathe in a relaxed manner with their eyes closed. Observe which hand moves first. The hand on the abdomen should rise first before the hand on the chest. This is the correct form of breathing known as diaphragmatic breathing (as mentioned earlier). The incorrect way of breathing, which is called chest breathing (or apical breathing), is where the hand on the chest elevates first. This may indicate a dysfunction with the Heart Sinew channels.

Assessment Two
The second assessment reflects the precise, delicate and sensitive nature of the channel movement in rotating and flexing. Ask the patient to simply bring their thumb and little finger together (a movement that is apparently unique to humans), and ask them to squeeze them together as you attempt to pull them apart with gentle force. The patient

should be able to keep the thumb and finger together comfortably without any discomfort. Pain and/or weakness indicates a dysfunction in the Heart Sinew channel.

Leg Jue Yin (Liver) Sinew channel

The Liver Sinew channels govern the movement of adduction of the legs, in addition to ensuring all major core movements are smooth and coordinated.

Note: The key to observing health of the Liver Sinew channel is that *all* body movements should be coordinated and carried out smoothly. It is the function of the Liver Sinew channel to connect to the centre of the body, from where all stable movement originates: 'Core stability gives good mobility'.

Key strength and engagement assessments of the Liver Sinew channel would be:

Assessment One

The first assessment of the Liver Sinew channel aims to check the strength and engagement of the patient's core, particularly in the region of the lower abdomen. Ask the patient to lie face up in a relaxed supine position, with their knees up and feet flat on the bed. With one arm, lift and support the patient's legs so that the upper legs are at 90 degrees to the bed, and the lower legs are in a horizontal position. Now, ask the patient to attempt to keep their legs in that position whilst you attempt to put the legs down. This should engage the Liver Sinew channel in the lower abdominal region, and the patient should be able to hold this position comfortably. If there is pain, discomfort or weakness, there may be a Liver Sinew channel dysfunction.

Assessment Two

The second assessment aims to check the patient's strength in adducting the lower limbs. Ask the patient to lie face up in a relaxed supine position and to abduct one leg to around 45 degrees whilst keeping the other leg straight and relaxed. Externally rotate the abducted leg slightly to engage the Liver Sinew channel, and place your hand on the medial aspect of the patient's ankle. Ask the patient to adduct the leg at a 45-degree angle (upwards and inwards) whilst you resist. Weakness or pain indicates a dysfunction with the Liver Sinew channel.

Arm Jue Yin (Pericardium) Sinew channel

The Pericardium Sinew channels govern the movement of adduction of the arms, engaging the diaphragm and enabling the breathing to be relaxed, and ensures all movement in the upper body is smooth and coordinated.

Note: The key to observing the Pericardium Sinew channel is that *all* body movement (especially of the upper limbs) should be coordinated and carried out smoothly. Like the Liver Sinew channel, it is the function of the Pericardium Sinew channel to connect to the centre of the body, from where all stable movement originates: 'Core stability gives good mobility'.

Key strength and engagement assessments of the Pericardium Sinew channel would be:

Assessment One

As with the Lung Sinew channel, the first assessment for the Pericardium Sinew channel should be to check the patient's breathing and engagement of the diaphragm. Ask the patient to lie in a relaxed supine position, and place one hand on the chest and the other on their abdomen. Allow the patient to breathe in a relaxed manner with their eyes closed. Observe which hand moves first. The hand on the abdomen should rise first before the hand on the chest. This is the correct form of breathing known as diaphragmatic breathing (as mentioned earlier). The incorrect way of breathing, which is called chest breathing (or apical breathing), is where the hand on the chest elevates first. This may indicate a dysfunction with the Pericardium Sinew channels.

Assessment Two

The second assessment checks the ability to draw the upper limbs inwards towards the chest. Ask the patient to lie face up in a relaxed supine position with their arms raised directly in front of them, with the middle fingers stretched upwards toward the ceiling. Place your hands on the inside of the patient's wrists and attempt to push their arms out to the side whilst the patient tries to resist. The patient should be able to comfortably hold their position. Pain and/or weakness indicates a dysfunction in the Pericardium Sinew channel.

Assessment Three

The third assessment checks the patient's ability to adduct their arms. Ask the patient to assume a standing position with their arms laterally abducted to around 30 degrees. Place your hand on the inside of their wrists and ask your patient to adduct their arms back to their sides whilst you resist. Pain, discomfort and/or weakness indicate a dysfunction in the Pericardium Sinew channel.

Chapter 7

Special Examinations

In Tui Na, special examinations cover assessments that are not necessarily Sinew channel or Chinese Medicine-specific, and mainly include orthopaedic and neuromuscular examinations that have been developed over years of clinical practice. Over the next few pages you will find key special examinations that are used to assess common conditions for key parts of the body.

The spine

Having a healthy spine is not only important in regards to the musculoskeletal system, flexibility and mobility, but also in regards to the health of the Zang Fu organs and internal bodily functions.

In Classical Chinese Medicine, the spine was known as the Celestial Pillar (Tian Zhu, 天柱), and connected Heaven (aspects of the mind) and Earth (the Jing and the Kidneys – essentially the foundation of the physical body). It is also thought to be the Celestial Pillar that transports Yang Qi to the rest of the body via the inner branches of the Bladder channel, and the Marrow (Sui, 髓) up through the spine to nourish the brain (known as the 'Sea of Marrow'). This shows the importance of the spine being healthy, with good mobility and flexibility, so that it can support the life and functioning of the rest of the body.

Natural curvatures of the spine

Without going into too much depth in regards to the anatomy of the spine (which can be found in any reputable anatomy and physiology publication), our spine can be split into four key parts:

- Cervical (made up of seven vertebrae, labelled C1-C7).

- Thoracic (made up of 12 vertebrae, labelled T1-T12).

- Lumbar (made up of 5 vertebrae, labelled L1-L5).

- Sacrum (made up of 5 *fused* vertebrae, labelled S1-S5).

Each part of the spine has a natural curve, which is present in order to help with structural alignment, flexibility and mobility of the spine. If the spine did not have a natural curve (and in some people, parts of it do not), the lack of flexibility and altered direction of force transfer would inevitably cause discomfort and potential damage.

The natural curves of the spine are known as lordosis, which curves anteriorly (concave), and kyphosis, which curves posteriorly (convex). In a healthy person, the cervical and lumbar vertebrae have a gentle lordotic curve, whereas the thoracic and sacral vertebrae have a gentle kyphotic curve.

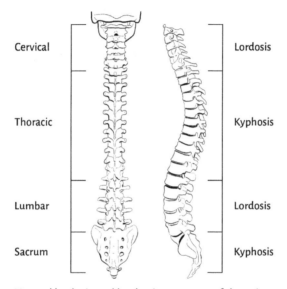

Cervical		Lordosis
Thoracic		Kyphosis
Lumbar		Lordosis
Sacrum		Kyphosis

Natural lordotic and kyphotic curvature of the spine

Although the spine should indeed have a natural curve in order to help with alignment, flexibility and force transfer, sometimes it may either have too much of a curve, or not enough of a curve. When this happens, we tend to label the spine as having lordosis or kyphosis (in terms of too much curvature) or as having a flat back (meaning the loss of natural curvature). These are discussed in more detail below.

Lordosis

When a patient is said to have lordosis, it means that their natural lordotic curve is excessive, affecting the cervical and lumbar vertebrae. It may also be known as hyperlordosis or 'hollow back'. When the spine has an excessive lumbar lordotic curve, it commonly causes the pelvis to tilt forwards, which in turn can affect the functioning of the internal organs.

Lordosis is often caused by weakness of the hamstrings and/or excessive tightness of the hip flexors, causing the pelvis to tilt forward and pull the lower spine out of alignment. Other causes include tightness in the lumbar area with weakness in the abdominal muscles, obesity and other disorders of the spine such as osteoporosis, spondylolisthesis and kyphosis elsewhere in the spine.

Kyphosis

When a patient is said to be in kyphosis, it means that their natural kyphotic curve is excessive, usually affecting the thoracic region of the spine. Patients with kyphosis have also been called 'hunch-backed' or 'hyperkyphotic'.

Kyphosis is often caused by poor posture, especially in later years, in addition to weakness of the Sinew channels of the back, congenital defects and bone diseases such as osteoporosis and spondylosis. A patient with moderate to severe kyphosis may also develop excessive lordosis in other regions of the spine in order to compensate for the angle of the spine.

Flat back

When a patient is said to have a 'flat back' it means that the spine has lost its natural curvature, resulting in the patient having what appears to be a flat back. It affects primarily the lumbar vertebrae, but can also affect the cervical and thoracic vertebrae. Having a 'flat back' will generally cause discomfort in the back due to reduced flexibility and mobility, and a change in force transfer. The lack of curve may also cause an imbalance of the spine, causing the patient to lean forward slightly or put their head forwards to compensate for balance. This puts further strain on the muscles. When the upper back is flat, it can especially affect mobility of the spine, in addition to the scapulae, which in turn may cause pain and discomfort in the shoulders.

A 'flat back' can be caused by shortening of the spine's anterior ligament (due to surgery or degenerative disc disease), compression fractures or ankylosing spondylitis.

Scoliosis

Although the spine naturally curves anteriorly (lordosis) and posteriorly (kyphosis), it should be straight in regards to laterally – that is, the spine should not have any sideways curvature. If the spine does develop a sideways curve one way or another, it is known as scoliosis. Scoliosis can be caused by a number of factors, including congenital birth defects, neurological or muscular conditions or injuries to the spine.

From a Chinese Medicine perspective, scoliosis is generally considered to be an imbalance of Yin and Yang (deficiency and excess) of the tissues supporting the spine. It is considered that the body is in excess at regions where the spine is being pulled to, and deficient in regions where the spine is being pulled away from (see the illustration above). Treatment should be designed at balancing the Yin and Yang regions by using tonifying or reducing methods (discussed in Section 1).

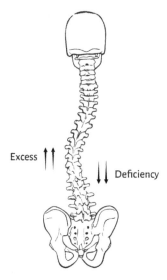

Scoliosis of the spine

Passive movement of the head and neck

Passive movement of the head and neck is a simple procedure to assess the structures of the cervical spine. When performing passive movement of the neck, in addition to pain of the Sinew channels, we are looking for certain red flags (essentially warning signs), which are known as the *Five Ds* and the *Three Ns* – these are dizziness, diplopia (double vision), dysphagia (difficulty swallowing), dysarthria (difficult speech), drop attack, nystagmus, nausea and neurological symptoms.

It is also possible to identify which nerve has been affected by asking the patient where they feel the neurological signs. The nerve that affects the index finger and thumb is the C6 nerve (emerging from below the C5 vertebra); the nerve that affects the middle finger is the C7 nerve (emerging from below the C6 vertebra); the nerve that affects the fourth and fifth fingers is the C8 nerve (emerging from below the C7 vertebra).

The Five Ds	The Three Ns
Dizziness	
Diplopia (double vision)	Nystagmus
Dysphagia (difficulty swallowing)	Nausea (and/or vomiting)
Dysarthria (difficult speech)	Neurological symptoms
Drop attack	

To perform passive movement of the head and neck, ask the patient to be in a seated position. Place one of your hands on top of the patient's head, and use your other hand to grasp the nape of their neck so that you can feel and palpate the spine and the soft tissues. Then, using the hand placed on the vertex of the head, perform a variety of gentle movements with the head, going through movements such as rotation, flexion, extension and lateral bends. All movement should be within the patient's natural anatomical range, and nothing should be forced. If any of the red flags mentioned above are made worse under gentle passive movement, the assessment should be stopped and the patient should be referred to their GP for further examination and imaging.

Neck compression test and the vertex knocking test

The neck compression test is a method that is done to assess nerve root pain, and to test for a compression of the nerve root within the cervical vertebrae at the cervical foramen. This test should only be done after passive movement of the neck has not given any significant signs, and there are no positive signs for the Five Ds or Three Ns (see above).

With the patient in a seated position, place both hands on to the vertex of the patient's head. Position the head into slight extension and side flexion to the side on which the patient is experiencing symptoms. Apply progressive yet gentle compression directly downwards through the spine. A positive sign would give rise to pain that originates from the neck and radiates down the limb to the affected side.

If there are no significant signs produced by causing compression, a 'vertex knock' can be applied in the same position. Instead of progressively applying pressure to the vertex, place one hand on top of the vertex, and knock the top of the head with the other hand (striking your own hand to reduce discomfort). This will send a shock through the spine that is slightly more forceful than using compression. Again, a positive sign would give rise to pain that originates from the neck and radiates down the limb to the affected side.

Neck flexion test

The neck flexion test is a simple method to assess nerve root damage or compression, commonly in the lumbar area. It is often used to confirm the diagnosis of lumbar disc herniation.

Ask the patient to lie on their back, in a relaxed supine position. Place one of your hands behind the occiput of the patient's head, and place the other hand on the patient's chest. Lift the patient's head so that their chin moves towards their chest as if they are looking down. This should cause the spinal cord to rise up to 2cm within the spinal canal, pulling on the nerve roots. If there is injury or compression of the nerve roots, the patient will feel pain and their symptoms will become worse.

Brachial plexus traction test

The brachial plexus traction test is used to rule out any damage or compression to the brachial plexus that may be causing neurological symptoms such as weakness, numbness or pain along the patient's arm to the associated side.

To perform the brachial plexus traction test, ask the patient to take a seated position and position their head slightly forward (no more than 30 degrees). Laterally tilt the patient's head slightly away from the affected side whilst taking hold of the patient's wrist of the affected side and pulling in the opposite direction. This should create a stretch along the Sinew channels with the focus around the brachial plexus region. A positive sign would be reproduction or worsening of the radiating symptoms down the affected arm, indicating injury or compression of the brachial plexus.

Iliac crest compression test

The iliac crest compression test is used to assess potential sacroiliac joint dysfunction, or a possible pelvic fracture. This test can be performed in two ways:

- With the patient lying on their back in a supine position, place one hand on each of the anterior iliac crests. Then, by applying pressure inwards on the two anterior iliac crests, create compression within the pelvis. If there is pain or discomfort in the pelvis, the test is positive, and may indicate a possible injury to the sacroiliac joint and/or a pelvic fracture.

- With the patient lying on their side in a recovery position, place one or two hands on the upper iliac crest and apply firm downward pressure, thus causing compression within the pelvis. Again, if there is pain or discomfort in the pelvis, the test is positive, and may indicate a possible injury to the sacroiliac joint and/or a pelvic fracture.

Pelvic separation test

Like the pelvic compression test mentioned above, the pelvic separation test is used to assess potential sacroiliac joint dysfunction, or a possible pelvic fracture. With the patient lying on their back in a supine position, place one hand on each of the anterior iliac crests. Then apply pressure downwards and outwards, separating the two iliac crests. If there is pain or discomfort in the pelvis, this shows a positive test and may indicate a possible injury to the sacroiliac joint and/or a pelvic fracture.

Heel to buttock test

The heel to buttock test is a simple assessment that can be used to determine a femoral nerve root compression, or strain of the iliopsoas muscle. With the patient lying comfortably on their front in prone position, place one hand on their lower back (for support), and take hold of the patient's ankle of the affected side with your other hand. Passively flex the patient's knee by quickly (but not forcefully) moving the ankle towards the patient's contralateral buttock. A reproduction of pain or discomfort in this position indicates femoral nerve root compression. To check for a possible iliopsoas strain, whilst keeping the ankle towards the buttock, lift the knee of the affected side to create extension of the hip – reproduction of pain will again suggest femoral nerve root compression and/or iliopsoas strain.

Upper extremities

There is a saying in Chinese Medicine that the 'shoulders are the gateway to the elbows, and the elbows are the gateways to the wrists'.

Drop arm test

The drop arm test is often used to confirm a supraspinatus and infraspinatus rupture. After palpating the shoulder, specifically at the infraspinatus and supraspinatus, ask the patient to sit or stand, and to passively abduct the affected arm to 90 degrees. Once in position, take away any support and ask the patient to hold their arm in position before asking them to slowly lower the arm back down to their side. If the patient is able to both hold their arm out to the side and then lower it in a controlled manner, the test is negative. If the patient is unable to hold the position, or if there is weakness and lack of control during the lower of the arm, the test is positive and it may suggest that there is an injury to the supraspinatus or infraspinatus muscles.

Internal rotation test

The internal rotation test of the shoulder is a commonly used test for sub-acromial impingement or injury to the supraspinatus tendon.

To perform the test, your patient should be seated. Elevate the patient's arm to 90 degrees in forward flexion, and support the elbow with one hand. Hold the patient's wrist with your other hand, and perform passive internal rotation by pulling the wrist down whilst holding the elbow in place. If the patient has pain or discomfort during the test, it suggests that there may be a sub-acromial impingement or a supraspinatus tear (to rule out a supraspinatus tear, perform the drop arm test).

Tennis elbow (lateral epicondylitis) test

While palpating the lateral epicondyle, have the patient hold their arm out with their elbow tucked into their side. Pronate the forearm so that the Yang channels are facing upwards, and flex the wrist forward comfortably so that the hand is vertical. To perform the test, extend the arm in this position at the elbow whilst it is still tucked into the side of the patient. As the arm is pronated and the wrist is already flexed, this should put a gentle stretch along the Yang channels of the arm. A positive test is if pain occurs over the lateral epicondyle, in the region of LI-11 (Qu Chi), indicating tennis elbow (lateral epicondylitis).

Golfer's elbow (medial epicondylitis) test

While palpating the medial epicondyle, have the patient hold their arm out with their elbow tucked into their side. Supinate the forearm so that the Yin channels are facing upwards, and extend the wrist back comfortably. To perform the test, extend the arm at the elbow whilst it is still tucked into the side of the patient. As the arm is supinated and the wrist is already extended, this should put a gentle stretch along the Yin channels. A positive test is if pain occurs over the medial epicondyle, in the region of H-3 (Shao Hai), indicating golfer's elbow (medial epicondylitis).

Wrist flexion test

The wrist flexion test is a very simple test to indicate the presence of carpal tunnel syndrome. To perform the test, take hold of the hand and flex the wrist as much as anatomically possible, causing an extension of the Yang channels. If the patient experiences an increase in numbness and/or pain, the sign is positive and suggests that the patient may have carpal tunnel syndrome.

Wrist triangular cartilage test

The triangular cartilage of the wrist helps towards stabilisation and rotation, and is load-bearing. To test for injury of the triangular cartilage, ask the patient to hold out their arm with their palms facing in a neutral plane. Take hold of the patient's hand at the fingers with one hand, and support the forearm below the wrist with the other hand. Bring the hand into ulna deviation, causing compression at the ulnocarpal joint on the triangular cartilage. A positive sign will elicit pain at the ulnar aspect of the wrist, indicating damage to the triangular cartilage.

Lower extremities

As with the upper extremities, there is a saying in Chinese Medicine that 'the hips are the gateways to the knees, and the knees are the gateways to the ankles'. Conversely, due to our lower extremities being weight-bearing, the ankles are considered to be the foundations to the knees, which are also the foundations to the hips and lower back.

Leg length inequality (pelvic alignment)

Leg length inequality can be due to three main factors: actual bone length differences; compaction of the femur into the hip joint; or pelvic misalignment. Although all three are possible, leg length inequality is most commonly due to the latter.

To check alignment of the pelvis, ask the patient to lie on their back in a relaxed supine position. Ask them to bring their knees up with their feet together on the bed, then to lift their hips up off the bed and then down again. This should put their pelvis into a position that their body *believes* is neutral. Then take their ankles, and lay the legs flat on the bed. It is now important to make three observations to check for pelvic alignment:

1. Place your thumbs on each of the medial malleoli to check if they are level.

2. Place your hands on both greater trochanters to check if they are level.

3. Place your hands at the top of the anterior iliac crest to check if they are level.

If (1) *alone* is not level, there is a possibility of a difference in actual leg length. If (2) is also not level, then the difference in leg length is likely to be due to either a compaction of the hip or misalignment of the pelvis. If (3) is not level, the leg length inequality is likely due to the pelvis being misaligned and that the actual legs are indeed the same length and the hip is not compacted.

It is important that all three checks are made, so that each factor can be either confirmed or dismissed. Once it has been confirmed what is causing the leg length inequality, treatment can be focused toward correcting the issue.

Knocking heel test (for the hip)

The knocking heel test is used when there is pain radiating down the leg, and we want to rule out any disorder of the hip joint. Ask the patient to lie in a relaxed supine position, and lift the affected leg to around 30 degrees with one hand, and then knock the heel perpendicularly (in the direction of the hip). The knock on the heel will send a shock wave up the leg and into the hip. If there is a hip disorder, the patient will experience sudden pain or discomfort.

Straight leg raise test (with flexion of the foot)

The straight let raise test is often used to test for any nerve root damage or compression to the nerves in the lumbar region, for example, due to possible disc herniation. The test should be done on both legs for comparison, and is usually performed on the good leg first, as a control.

Ask the patient to lie on their back in a relaxed supine position. With them lying flat, take one leg and raise it slowly whilst keeping it completely straight. Once the patient feels discomfort or pain, do not raise the leg any further. Lower the leg slightly, until the pain or discomfort disappears, and quickly perform dorsiflexion of the foot – this will eliminate the possibility of the discomfort or pain initially experienced being due to hamstring or iliotibial tract tightness. If there is pain in the lower back, this suggests a positive sign for nerve root compression that is potentially due to lumbar disc herniation, as the dorsiflexion has pulled on and created tension in the sciatic nerve.

Note: If there is indeed compression to the nerve root, it is highly unlikely that the patient will be comfortable having their leg raised beyond 60 degrees from the treatment couch. Limited mobility in this test is also a positive sign.

Figure of four test

The figure of four test is used to find pathologies of the hip, pelvis and lower back. The position allows the lower limb to combine the three movements of *flexion*, *abduction* and *external rotation*, enabling assessment of the hip and sacroiliac joint.

To perform the figure of four test, ask the patient to lie on their back in a supine position. Place the patient's affected leg in a figure of four position (with the hip flexed and abducted with the ankle placed just above the knee of the opposite leg). Whilst stabilising the pelvis, gentle force should be directed posteriorly onto the knee that is bent, slowly moving through a normal anatomical range of movement. A positive test will elicit pain if there is a presence of a hip or sacroiliac joint pathology.

Lateral/medial collateral ligament test

To perform the test for lateral collateral ligament, ask the patient to lie in a relaxed supine position, and hold their affected leg so that it has a slight bend at the knee (the knee should not be locked straight, but also not be fully bent). Place one hand just above the medial joint line of the knee, and the other hand just above the lateral side of the ankle. Initiate a gentle pull with the hand by the knee, and a gentle push with the hand just above the ankle. This should cause the lateral side of the knee joint to open slightly. A positive test would elicit pain if there is a ligament injury or tear, or pain and abnormal movement if the ligament is completely torn. Injury to the ligament can also be confirmed with the addition of palpation at the injury site.

To perform the test for medial collateral ligament, ask the patient to lie in a relaxed supine position, and hold their affected leg so that it has a slight bend at the knee (the knee should not be locked straight, but also not be fully bent). Place one hand just above the lateral joint line of the knee, and the other hand just above the medial side of the ankle. Initiate a gentle push with the hand by the knee, and a gentle pull with the hand just above the ankle. This should cause the medial side of the knee joint to open slightly. A positive test would elicit pain if there is a ligament injury or tear, or pain and abnormal movement if the ligament is completely torn. Injury to the ligament can also be confirmed with the addition of palpation at the injury site.

Anterior/posterior cruciate ligament test

The anterior/posterior cruciate ligament tests are two of the most common assessments used on the knee, and are easy to perform, assessing the stability and structures of the anterior and posterior cruciate ligaments.

To perform the test for the anterior cruciate ligament (ACL), ask the patient to lie on their back in a supine position with the affected knee bent to around 90 degrees. Slightly sit on the patient's feet with the side of your thigh, and place each thumb on EX-LE-5 (Xi Yan) with the hands wrapped around the calf. From this position, pull the tibia towards you to assess the distance of travel and also the feeling of the travel coming to its end point. If the travel is excessive, and/or the end point comes to a soft halt, then there is damage to the ACL. If the travel is minimal, and the end point comes to a sudden halt, then the ACL is intact. This test should be repeated on both knees for comparison.

To perform the test for the posterior cruciate ligament (PCL), both patient and practitioner should be in the same position. With the hands placed on the knee, again in the same position, push the tibia posteriorly to assess distance of travel and also the feeling of the travel coming to its end point. If the travel is excessive and/or the end point comes to a soft halt, there is damage to the PCL. If the travel is minimal, and the end point comes to a sudden halt, the PCL is intact. This test should be repeated on both knees for comparison.

Menisci tear test

To perform assessment of the medial menisci of the knee joint, ask the patient to lie in a relaxed supine position and to fully flex the knee. Place one hand on the knee, palpating the postero-medial aspect of the knee joint, and use the other hand to lift the foot and hold the heel of the foot. Rotate the ankle internally, then perform Yao Fa in an external direction by making large circles with the foot to cause slight rotation, flexion and extension of the knee.

To perform assessment of the lateral menisci of the knee joint, again ask the patient to lie in a relaxed supine position, and to fully flex the knee. Place one hand on the knee, palpating the postero-lateral aspect of the knee joint, and use the other hand to lift the foot and hold the heel. Rotate the ankle externally, then perform Yao Fa in an internal direction by making large circles with the foot to cause slight rotation, flexion and extension of the knee.

In both assessments, a positive sign would elicit pain localised to the menisci, and a grinding or clicking sound in the knee. To further confirm menisci damage, the patient should be asked if the knee either locks up or gives way on a regular basis.

HAND TECHNIQUES

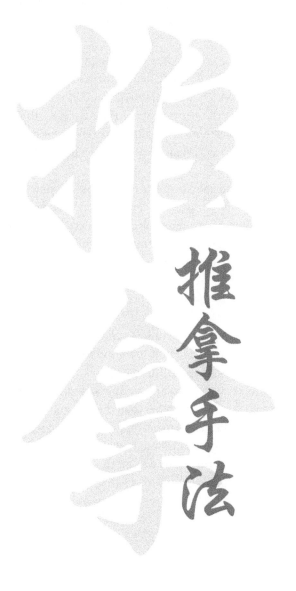

Chapter 8

Introduction to Tui Na Techniques

This section of the book has been written really to accompany a face-to-face Tui Na teaching programme, or to serve as a reminder for those who have already learned the techniques of Tui Na. This is largely due to the fact that it is impossible to effectively learn the postures, body shape and practical movements of Tui Na simply from a book or a video.

When learning Tui Na techniques, it is not enough to simply learn the movements. Each Tui Na technique has a function, and a specific reason to be used – just like different tools in a tool box. It is necessary to understand the functions and roles of each technique, so that the correct technique can be used at the right time, on the right patient and for the right reason. Try to understand the nature of each technique by feeling what it is doing to the patient, and also experience it yourself by having treatment from another student or practitioner.

Some techniques work on specific parts of the body, where others may not. Some techniques may feel more comfortable on certain body shapes, where others may not. This is why it is important to have a repertoire of a variety of techniques so that you can be adaptable and spontaneous in your treatment. Furthermore, practise each technique at different angles and in different positions around the patient. In clinical practice, it is useful to be able to quickly adapt to different scenarios. It is not good if you are only able to perform a certain technique in one position, and then you get a patient who is unable to assume that position!

When studying and learning each technique, and indeed during clinical practice once you have become a Tui Na practitioner, it is a good idea to apply the act of Ting (聽) that was introduced in the first chapter. This will help focus your awareness, so that you remain entirely mindful of your hand and body movements – attempt to make each movement more relaxed and even smoother than the last, and travel to the most efficient depth. This will allow the hand shapes to become natural, and feel more comfortable for both you and your patient. Progression should never stop. Once the movements become coordinated and connected to the body, we can then begin to add what are known as the Five Virtues of Tui Na, and begin to internalise the energetics of what each hand technique is designed to do.

Open your eyes!

A common mistake for many bodywork therapists, especially those who follow older traditions, is closing the eyes whilst working in the hope that it will increase their sensitivity by 'disabling' one of the senses.

First, although the loss of a sense may heighten other senses over some time, this would not happen immediately simply by closing the eyes for a few seconds. What's more, closing the eyes sets up a series of triggers that directs the Qi, Shen, and therefore our awareness inwards towards our own consciousness. This is why closing the eyes should be reserved for sleeping or self-cultivation exercises such as meditation and some aspects of Qi Gong. During treatment we want to guide our awareness out of our own body, through our extremities and out into the patient in order to feel what is happening within the patient. We must therefore keep our eyes open and focused on what we are doing.

The Five Virtues of Tui Na

The Five Virtues of Tui Na are essentially the minimum requirements that a practitioner should be able to apply to each technique. When performing each technique, whether it is a hand technique, stretch or joint manipulation, the practitioner should keep in mind each of the Five Virtues. Classically it was considered that a student had only attained Gong (功, skill) once all of the Five Virtues had been achieved and internalised. It was then important for the student who became a doctor to keep in mind the Five Virtues during further practice and during each treatment, and aim to increase their skill further. When practising and when in treatment, the practitioner should still strive to apply each of the Five Virtues to each and every technique that they do. By adhering to the Five Virtues of Tui Na, the practitioner can ensure that their techniques are efficient and effective in treatment.

The Five Virtues

The Five Virtues are continuous, powerful, even, soft and deep. Classically it was considered that a practitioner had only attained *Gong* (功, *skill*) once all of the *Five Virtues* had been properly *achieved* and *internalised*.

Continuously and lasting (持久)

Unlike many other bodywork therapies, Tui Na contains techniques that are often performed for long periods of time at the same location on the body. It is this endurance that ensures that the technique indeed reaches the area and level of dysfunction, without simply forcing its way in. When performing a technique, in particular the basic hand techniques, the practitioner should have the ability to do so for long periods of time without loss of quality. If a condition is located within the deeper layers of the body, it is the endurance of the technique that will enable the practitioner to reach the desired level of the body in order to affect the dysfunctional layer.

One of the key principles of being able to perform a technique for long periods of time is the relaxation of the practitioner and the efficiency of the body and structure. By ensuring that the muscles are engaged just enough as they need to be, and that the body structure and posture is aligned in order to transfer power rather than store it, the practitioner should be able to perform each technique for maximum periods of time with minimal effort. Eliminating any unnecessary tension is essential in having endurance for each technique.

Powerfully and strongly (有力)

A Tui Na practitioner should be able to apply their techniques powerfully and vigorously. In order to make a change to the body's tissues, there needs to be enough strength behind a technique to enable this change. However, although Tui Na therapy can indeed feel strong and at times uncomfortable, which it should, it is vitally important to distinguish the difference between power and force. Being able to apply the appropriate amount of pressure based on the patient's age, constitution and body part/area is important. Many practitioners will mistake a forceful massage for being a good massage. Pain during treatment does not mean beneficial. The feeling after a forceful massage, other than the relief that it is now over, is mainly a consequence of the release of chemicals within the body such as endorphins, adrenaline and adenosine that cause the feeling of euphoria and pain relief. This should not be mistaken for feeling better, as it is simply a reaction to the pain and discomfort caused during treatment.

Issuing power through a technique rather than force can again only be done through relaxation. By being relaxed and transferring power into a technique, the practitioner can have increased awareness and alter the amount of pressure and strength directed into the patient. Applying the correct pressure is discussed in more detail below.

Evenly and uniformly (均匀)

Rather than the relaxing, sweeping movements of certain forms of massage such as Swedish or Western remedial massage, Tui Na has been known to be described as a bit of a pummelling. However, if performed correctly, the rhythmic compressions of Tui Na can indeed induce relaxing and almost hypnotic effects on the body.

The virtue of performing techniques evenly and uniformly refers to the ability to maintain an even rhythm of pressure and tempo. Techniques should not be performed erratically, as this can prevent the patient from being able to relax the mind as it attempts to predict what will happen next. When techniques are done in a rhythmical fashion, the body can attenuate to the movement and the mind can begin to relax. This will allow further relaxation of the tissues, therefore allowing deeper massage if required.

When training in China, more specifically within the larger hospitals and universities such as Shanghai, students are required to perform certain techniques onto a pad that is hooked up to a computer that measures and records the speed and pressure of the manipulations or techniques. This method, along with feedback from fellow students and teachers, gives the student a visual guide to the evenness of their technique. Students are encouraged to produce smooth and rhythmical readings as opposed to erratic and jagged readings.

Softly and gently (柔和)

Being soft or gentle does not refer to a lack of power but to being able to manipulate with ease as opposed to aggressive force. Again, referring to the ability to avoid *force*, changes should be able to happen with ease. This will be the case if the Sinew channels have sufficiently been opened before using techniques that require more strength.

If, as a practitioner, I took hold of your arm in a sharp and aggressive way, ready to manipulate a joint or perform traction, you will naturally tense up and resist due to your body feeling that there is a threat. This is going to make it much more difficult for me to create space in the joint, as the tissues will prevent any movement. However, if I took hold of your arm in a gentle and relaxed manner, your body would feel no threat and allow me to gently create traction on the joint.

You may have experienced or witnessed some practitioners (of Tui Na or other bodywork therapies) using brute force in order to perform a spinal adjustment or joint mobilisation. This simply is not necessary, and although there are exceptions to every rule, should generally be avoided.

Thoroughly and deeply (深透)

Although we have discussed the mistake of going too deep, it can also be the case that the practitioner does not penetrate deeply enough. Many practitioners will only work on the surface of the body and not manage to alter the state of the tissues at a deeper level. Although some techniques *should* be performed at the Pi Fu (skin) and Wei Qi layer, most Tui Na techniques are required to work on the Jing Jin (Sinew channels) later. Therefore, this virtue refers to the ability of achieving the desired depth of treatment.

The Five Virtues of Tui Na	
Continuously/lasting (持久)	Being able to continuously perform a single technique
Powerfully/strongly (有力)	Being able to apply the appropriate amount of pressure based on the patient's age, constitution and body part/area; using power as opposed to force
Evenly/uniformly (均匀)	Being able to maintain an even rhythm of pressure and tempo
Softly/gently (柔和)	Being able to manipulate with ease as opposed to aggressive or abrasive force
Thoroughly/deeply (深透)	Being able to achieve the desired depth of treatment

Shaping the body's landscape

Learning how to touch and palpate sensitively and effectively is vital when working with the body. It is our only way of directly analysing what is going on beneath the skin. When palpating many different bodies, over time our sense of touch through the fingers, hands and nervous system becomes more and more sensitive, and remembers things that our brain does not. Our hands essentially become experts in anatomy, subconsciously comparing and cross-referencing against the many bodies that have been palpated previously, and analysing what is perceived as either normal and abnormal.

Palpation

Our hands become *experts* in *anatomy,* remembering things that our brain does not.

As is the case in many of the Chinese Arts, in Tui Na the body is viewed as a 'landscape'. The shape and musculature of the body form the mountains, valleys and the caves, and the joints are considered to be the wells, springs, rivers and seas (as such, the five Shu points). The Primary channels are considered to be the waterways, whilst the Sinew channels are seen as the river beds, and the acupuncture points are seen as being the temples or caves. As Tui Na practitioners, we are interested in three main landforms: mountains, valleys and caves.

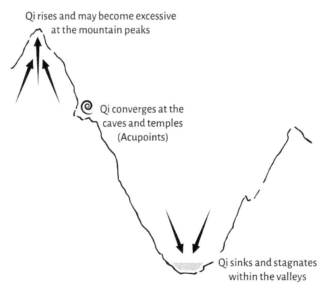

Qi rises and may become excessive at the mountain peaks

Qi converges at the caves and temples (Acupoints)

Qi sinks and stagnates within the valleys

The nature of Qi within the landscape

- Mountains: The mountains of the body are the peaks and apexes of the muscles – they are considered to be the muscular 'bumps'. It is at the mountains of the body that the Qi rises and collects at the top. Due to the fact that Qi rises to the top of the mountains, it is at the muscle apexes that tissues are likely to become too Yang, and are therefore more likely suffer from being excess. Essentially it is within these areas that the body is prone to tightness, tension and hypertonicity.

- Valleys: The valleys of the body are where the depressions lie within the muscles, tissue fibres and joints. It is within the valleys of the tissues that the Qi, Blood and Body Fluids sink and descend, and collect at the bottom. Due to the fact that the Qi, Blood and Body Fluids descend into the valleys, it is within the depressions of the body that stagnation or stasis is most likely to occur, and the Vital Substances become stuck and cannot move. It is also within the valleys that the tissues are more likely to become empty and deficient.

- Caves: The caves of the body are small hole like depressions, again within the superficial muscles and tissues fibres. It is within these small depressions that the Qi swirls and converges, and are most likely to be active acupuncture points that the Primary channels pass through. The caves are the depressions that we are looking for when palpating for specific acupuncture points. Due to the fact that Qi converges at these points, there is often stagnation, which is one reason why acupuncture points are often tender or sensitive to touch. However, because the Qi within these caves is more 'active' than that of the Qi within the valleys, it is easier to resolve stagnation and encourage the flow of Qi through the channel.

When we first lay our hands on a patient, the true 'landforms' of the body may be difficult to palpate at first. This is due to both a lack of sensitivity of the practitioner, and also a layer of 'sediment' that lies over the tissues due to stagnations and swellings. This layer of sediment lies over the tissues like a thick blanket, making them difficult to feel and work with. Before any diagnosis or treatment takes place, we first need to 'shape' the body's landscape and work through this layer of sediment, stagnation and swelling, with a sensitivity of touch that needs to be deep enough to move, yet soft enough to not cause damage (more information on applying the correct pressure can be found on the next page). This allows us to unearth the true contours of the body tissues, and to see and feel what is truly happening with the body's musculature.

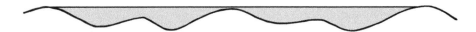

Layer of 'sediment' and 'tension' lying over the body's landscape

The way that we remove the sediment that lies over the tissues is first of all by putting our hands on the patient's body and just *feeling*. Use techniques such as **Mo Fa, Tui Fa** and **An Fa** to press and feel what is going on under your hands. This allows us to work out what is actually the musculature of the body, and what is the sediment, stagnation and the excesses or deficiencies. Begin with using techniques lightly enough to not affect the tissues, but strongly enough to move the sediment. Slowly increase the pressure and depth little by little whilst sliding your hands over the tissues and feeling for the body's landforms. At first you may only feel a smooth surface, although over the space of a few minutes, the body's true structures will begin to emerge and what you will feel are the true contours of the body; it will feel as if you are sculpting a landscape.

It is important to remember that this process of preparing and palpating the body is just a beginning process, and it is not necessarily therapeutic. However, by the very nature of doing something to the patient's body, their tissues will react and change shape. This alone will help the body to become more reactive to the treatment that is to follow.

Shaping the body's landscape

The three main *landforms* (formed by the *musculature* of the body) that we look at in Tui Na are the *mountains, valleys* and *caves*.

Applying the correct pressure during treatment

Although Tui Na is generally considered a 'deep' or 'strong' therapy, it should not mean that the practitioner causes unnecessary discomfort to the patient. As stated previously within the Five Virtues of Tui Na, techniques should be powerful (but not forceful), soft (without tension) and deep (meaning deep enough to have an influential impact). Techniques should also be practised gently with little pressure until good technique and hand positioning has been achieved. This is to avoid any injury to the practitioner as well as to the patient (or volunteer). Once the technique is good enough, more pressure can be applied (according to the patient's constitution/condition).

Transformation

The most efficient *transformation* occurs at the *boundary of change* – the border between *relaxed* and *contracted* tissue.

As with anything in life, the most efficient transformation will happen at the boundary between two different states. For example, within the practice of Tui Na, the body is most likely to respond to change when working at the level of the border between relaxed tissue and contracted tissue. If the pressure is too light, very little change will occur; if the pressure is too strong, the body will react in an adverse way and likely cause pain to the patient. This may feel beneficial temporarily due to the body's reaction to pain, although it is unlikely to benefit the patient in the long run, and is likely to slow down healing due to the body having to repair unnecessarily damaged tissue.

It is important, especially whilst learning a bodywork therapy, but also when in practice, to always ask for patient feedback during the treatment. This is to help gauge your pressure and also to put the patient at ease, knowing that you are taking their experience into account. There is a fine line between therapeutic discomfort (or tenderness) and pain. Tenderness is okay, whereas pain is counterproductive – the body tissues will respond by attempting to protect the body and tightening up (as they are designed to!).

Powerful yet relaxed

If you are *tense* in your techniques, the patient's body will give you *tension* back. If you are *relaxed*, so will the patient be – the patient's body will essentially mimic what you do.

Reactivity of fascia

As Tui Na practitioners, it is vital we gain some understanding of the fascial system and the implications of certain techniques on the various types of fascial tissue. Working the fascial tissue can decrease Qi and Blood stagnation, and improve the free flow of Qi and Blood to certain areas. Within Chinese Medicine, it is thought that the fascia system comes under the category of the Huang (肓, membranes), which essentially bridge the gap between the Qi and the Sinew channels – the Qi nourishes the Huang, which in turn nourishes and strengthens the Sinew channels.

Fascial tissue is extremely susceptible to stimulation, and is highly sensory loaded – even more so than our spine. It should also move smoothly and glide freely over the tissues. When it loses this ability, it also loses the ability to transmit force or Qi throughout the body. As Tui Na practitioners, it is hugely important to understand the different types of pressure that effect fascia. As fascia is highly sensory and can sit closely to the skin, we don't need to go too hard or cause the patient pain or discomfort through pressure. This will simply push the body or central nervous system into threat mode, causing tension so that the body can protect itself. When this happens, there will be more stagnation that will impair the body's ability to heal and move correctly. Stimulating fascia in the correct way, however, enables us to 'convince' the body and nervous system to let us move past the fascia, and deeper into the Sinew channels where we can begin to be firmer with our technique. As the body feels safer in its environment because we 'eased' into the tissues, it will let us move with greater ease and strength, thus enabling better flow of Qi and Blood. This is why in Tui Na we have the different stages of treatment (discussed in Chapter 10), and it is vitally important that we work with the opening stage, the treatment stage and the closing stage. Again, this is a lesson in sensitivity and subtlety, rather than rushing in hard and fast.

The six basic technique categories

Within Tui Na, there are two types of manipulation and technique. One type of manipulation is called single, or simple, manipulation, and the other type is called complex manipulation – not because it is harder or more difficult to perform, but because it contains a number of different movements that may be used in different ways.

Classically, all Tui Na techniques within the simple type were placed into one of six categories depending on the movement and principles behind them or their therapeutic effect. All techniques within each category have similar core movements, with just the hand shape or positioning being different. Although these categories vary from school to school, the six technique categories are generally considered to be *swaying*, *rubbing*, *vibrating and shaking*, *pressing*, *striking*, and *passive joint manipulation*. Some schools may consider Qi emission (Wai Qi Liao Fa, 外氣療法) or bone setting (Zheng Gu, 正骨) as separate categories, although they may also come under vibrating and passive joint movement categories respectively.

Swaying (摆动类)

The swaying category is quite possibly the most difficult category of techniques due to seemingly awkward and unnatural types of movement that should be carried out to make each technique effective. Movement of each hand technique within this category comes from the shoulder and a swaying or swing-type movement of the whole arm, with emphasis on swaying the forearm.

This category is considered to be one of the most important categories in that the techniques can enable the practitioner to understand how to transfer power through structure and posture rather than using muscular force.

Techniques that belong to the swaying category: Gun Fa, Yi Zhi Chan Tui Fa, Rou Fa

Rubbing (摩擦类)

Rubbing techniques are mostly used to release tissues, warm the area and remove stagnation of Qi and Blood. Techniques within this category are performed in either a circular or linear direction and vary in speeds depending on the desired therapeutic effect.

Techniques that belong to the rubbing category: Mo Fa, Tui Fa, Ca Fa, Ma Fa, Cuo Fa, Nian Fa

Vibrating and shaking (振动类)

Techniques within the vibrating category utilise vibration to move Qi and Blood and to remove stagnation. Vibrations are generally done at high frequency and low amplitude and focused on specific tissues, organs or joints. **Zhen Fa**, one of the techniques within this category, requires the use of quite advanced Nei Gong in order to achieve vibrational force travelling through the arm and palms/fingers; however, other techniques such as **Dou Fa** simply require the practitioner to shake using vibration of the muscles.

Techniques that belong to the vibrating and shaking category: Zhen Fa, Dou Fa

Pressing (按压类)

The pressing category contains techniques that apply static pressure on to specific areas of the body with the fingers, hands, forearms/elbows or knees in a perpendicular direction to the body tissue. These techniques often rely on the difference in force between application and release of pressure to facilitate the removal of stagnation and to regulate the flow of Qi and Blood. Pressure may be for very short or prolonged periods of time.

Techniques that belong to the pressing category: An Fa, Na Fa, Dian Fa, Tan Bo Fa, Si Fa, Nie Fa, Ya Fa

Striking (叩击类)

All techniques within the striking category require the practitioner to hit specific areas of the body at varying depths depending on the desired outcome. Techniques are usually used for dissipating Qi and removing stagnation, and are selected based on the depth of stagnation, whether it is on the exterior layers of the body or more internal.

Techniques that belong to the striking category: Pai Fa, Ji Fa

Passive joint manipulation (活动关节类)

Techniques within this category require the practitioner to go through a range of movement and manipulation exercises on specific joints, usually to mobilise or open up the spaces within the joints, or to stretch along the Sinew channels. For these techniques to be effective, the patient is required to be completely passive and relaxed so that the practitioner has total control over the joints and soft tissues, and can take the joints through their normal anatomical ranges and restore functional movement.

Techniques that belong to the passive joint manipulation category: Yao Fa, Ba Shen Fa, Ban Fa, Shen Zhan Fa

Category	Techniques
Swaying (摆动类)	Gun Fa – Rolling Yi Zhi Chan Tui Fa – Single finger meditation Rou Fa – Kneading
Rubbing (摩擦类)	Mo Fa – Circular rubbing Tui Fa – Pushing Ca Fa – To-and-fro rubbing Ma Fa – Wiping Cuo Fa – Palm twisting Nian Fa – Finger twisting
Vibrating and shaking (振动类)	Zhen Fa – Vibrating Dou Fa – Shaking

Category	Techniques
Pressing (按压类)	An Fa – Pressing Na Fa – Grasping Dian Fa – Striking Tan Bo Fa – Plucking Si Fa – Tearing Nie Fa – Pinching Ya Fa – Supressing
Striking (叩击类)	Pai Fa – Patting Ji Fa – Percussing
Passive joint manipulation (活动关节类)	Yao Fa – Rocking/rotating Ba Shen Fa – Traction/stretching Ban Fa – Pulling/twisting Shen Zhan Fa – Stretching/extending

Choosing and combining Tui Na techniques – prescription building

Manipulations and techniques can be combined in different ways, and just like when prescribing Herbal Medicine or choosing acupuncture points, diligent Tui Na students would be taught to use the *Jun Chen Zuo Shi* (君臣佐使, emperor, minister, assistant and servant) system of Chinese Medicine. This helps us to decide which manipulations or techniques are most important for the patient, and which manipulations or techniques can support the important ones. This is the classical view on how to put together your Tui Na treatment plan or prescription. Within modern Tui Na teachings, in both the East and the West, this concept is gradually fading away. Although still used widely in Chinese Herbal Medicine and Acupuncture, many Tui Na doctors will not use it, and those who do still use this method of technique prescribing do not share these methods until you have shown that you are a good student.

There are no specific techniques that are, for example, 'emperor' or 'minister' techniques – *any* technique can be classed as any of the four classifications. A technique's importance depends on the patient and the condition that they present with. For example, **Gun Fa** may be considered as an emperor technique for one patient, but as an assistant technique for another or a servant for another. It is essentially a hierarchy system used to demonstrate the importance of certain techniques for a specific patient, and the amount of focus and importance that each technique is given during any specific treatment.

If a patient presents with shoulder pain or neck pain, **Gun Fa** may be considered as an emperor technique, although you may not consider **Ma Fa** to be an important technique of choice. On the other hand, if you see a patient who presents with insomnia, **Gun Fa** may not be used at all, and **Yi Zhi Chan Tui Fa** or **Mo Fa** may be considered to be the emperor technique with **Ma Fa** to be a minister technique. So you can see that the importance of each technique can change, in the same way that there is no element that is most important within the Wu Xing theory, and each element can be more dominant/important at any one time.

When considering a patient prescription within Tui Na, it is important that you think about which techniques should be most important and which ones should assist and so on, especially during training, as this will help you to understand the function and importance of each technique within different conditions. It is interesting to see how a technique can be very important for one patient or condition, and not so much for another patient or condition. Over time you will see which techniques and manipulations are best used for certain conditions and diagnoses, and this helps to build your understanding.

Jun (君) emperor techniques

Jun (emperor) techniques are considered essential for the patient and should be the main techniques used for treatment as they will be the most effective. Examples of Jun (emperor) techniques might be **Ban Fa** to help with joint misalignments, **Ba Shen Fa** for opening and releasing compressions, **Pai Fa** to expel exterior Wind, **Ca Fa** to resolve stagnation, **Tan Bo Fa** to break down scar tissue and so on. Essentially any technique can be considered as the Jun (emperor) technique depending on the presenting condition, and techniques should be chosen according to the indication, and hopefully not chosen based on ease or convenience.

Chen (臣) minister techniques

Chen (minister) techniques have two functions. First, they are used to help the Jun (emperor) technique to treat the main cause of the condition, and second, they are used to treat any coexisting conditions that the patient has. This may be headaches that have been caused by neck or shoulder pain, for example. Although within Chinese Medicine it is essentially to treat the root cause, we still treat the symptoms as often these will gain relief quicker, and then the patient can have a better quality of life during the course of treatment.

Zuo (佐) assistant techniques

Zuo (assistant) techniques, like Chen (minister) techniques, are used to help the main techniques in order to treat the main cause of the condition. They are also used to help prepare the patient for the main techniques, such as using **Rou Fa** and **Tui Fa** to warm up the patient ready to perform **Ban Fa**, or perhaps using **Mo Fa** and **Gun Fa** to open up the channels before applying strong pressure with **An Fa** or **Ya Fa**.

Shi (使) servant techniques

Shi (servant) techniques are often those that have little to no therapeutic effect on the patient, but are used to increase the effectiveness of the other techniques, or to prevent the likelihood of any adverse effects caused by the main techniques. For example, after using a strong variation of **An Fa** on specific acupressure points or Ashi points, I may decide to use a dissipating technique such as **Ji Fa** or **Pai Fa** to resolve any stagnation that I have caused whilst using **An Fa**. This helps to prevent any soreness or prolonged stagnation in the area that may have occurred as a result of treatment.

Additionally, Shi (servant) techniques may be used to guide the Qi to various parts of the body. For instance, should I have a patient who presents with severe pain in the lower back, whilst I perform a technique such as **Gun Fa** to warm the area and attempt to warm and release the area, I may use **Yi Zhi Chan Tui Fa** on BL-57 or SI-11 in order to draw the Qi away from the lower back so that the patient feels less discomfort whilst I give treatment to the injured area.

Chapter 9

Tui Na Hand Techniques

The following pages cover the therapeutic actions and methods of the foundation hand techniques of Tui Na, referred to in Chinese as the Ji Ben Tui Na Shou Fa (基本推拿手法). As stated earlier in the book, this chapter should be used as a companion to entirely new students whilst studying on a hands-on practical course in Tui Na, or as a reminder to already qualified practitioners. The following Tui Na techniques are set out in alphabetical order, with the passive joint manipulation techniques placed at the end.

按法 An Fa (pressing)

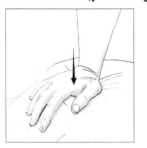

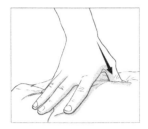

Technique category
Pressing

Stages of treatment
Treatment stage

Therapeutic actions
An Fa is a technique that is used to help relax muscles by causing a transition from Yang to Yin, and to help clear occlusions and stagnation by creating a pressure build-up to cause a resolve in stagnation. An Fa can also be used to activate Qi and Blood circulation within an area and to help increase Blood flow.

An Fa, meaning 'pressing technique', is one of the oldest techniques used within Chinese Massage, and can be seen as part of the names of older massage styles An Mo (pressing/rubbing) and An Qiao (pressing/stepping). It is one of the most fundamental techniques within Tui Na, and is a simple technique that is often used on acupressure points to activate a specific point or part of a channel, or used on Ashi points such as tensions and knots. It is used during the treatment stage, and is essentially used to help remove stagnation and obstructions within the channels. It does so by causing a build-up of pressure by temporarily blocking the flow of Qi and Blood. Once the pressure is released, Qi and Blood can flow through the channel with greater force, helping to remove any obstructions. Additionally, the increase in pressure and tension in the muscle and sinew fibres enables the Yang (tension) to become much greater so that it transforms to Yin (relaxation).

An Fa can be performed with the thumb, fingertips (known as Dian Fa), belly of the fingers, the palm, the forearm or two overlapped palms to press perpendicularly onto the body. It is used during the treatment stage once the body has been warmed up and the Sinew channels have been opened. The pressure exerted should increase steadily from light to heavy. Sudden violent force should be avoided as this can cause spasm of the muscle as the body tries to protect itself from trauma. This manipulation must not be performed over the spine or other bony prominences, and pressure is generally applied for only a few seconds at a time, especially if the pressure exerted is strong.

Method

An Fa may at first seem easy to perform; however, in order to perform the technique correctly, focus and care must be taken in the timing, pressure and structure of the technique.

- Locate a point on the body. This can be a specific acupuncture point, Ashi point or any other part of the body you would like to stimulate.

- As both you and the patient breathe out, apply pressure steadily with the thumb (or other parts of the hand or arm that are used to perform An Fa) perpendicularly on to the point, until you reach the desired depth. The depth should depend on the desired outcome, area of treatment and diagnosis of the patient.

- Keep a constant pressure on the point at the desired depth for a number of seconds (if firm) or up to a couple of minutes (if gentle).

- If you want to nourish the point, release the pressure slowly as both you and the patient breathe out. If you want to release spasm of the muscles or tissues that you are pressing, release the pressure quickly.

An Fa requires great sensitivity, and the pressure applied should depend on the level of the 'boundary of change', as discussed at the beginning of this chapter regarding applying the correct pressure. If the pressure is not firm enough, the effect will not be strong enough. However, if the pressure is too firm, then too much stagnation will be caused and the opposite desired effect will happen. Becoming sensitive to touch is essential when using An Fa.

Tips

- Line up your thumb or fingers with the forearm to create greater strength and structure.

- If the pressure required is relatively deep with a chance of discomfort to the patient, apply around 60 per cent pressure during the first breath, then apply the rest of the pressure on the second or third breath to allow the body to attenuate better.

Variations
压法 Ya Fa (supressing)

Some schools would consider the technique Ya Fa to be a variation of An Fa. It is essentially the same movement, which involves the practitioner pressing into the patient with a particular body part. Ya Fa is translated as 'supressing' or 'pressure technique', and is generally performed with the elbow or the forearm; it can also be done with the knees. It is more static than An Fa, and is performed stronger and for longer periods in order to penetrate to deeper levels of the larger muscle groups. For this reason, it is often used on areas of the body where there are larger and stronger muscles groups, such as the Bladder Sinew channel.

A variation of Ya Fa is to apply pressure perpendicularly into the body with the elbow as normal, increasing pressure slowly. Once the technique has reached the desired depth, hold the pressure for a few seconds whilst shaking the hand in a relaxed manner (as if shaking water off the hand). This will cause vibrations to travel from the hand to the elbow, and into the patient's body, helping the relaxation of the soft tissues.

按压复位法 An Ya Fu Wei Fa (press and supress to reset)

An Ya Fu Wei Fa, means 'to press and supress to reset', meaning to reset a locked joint using pressure. This variation of An Fa is classed in the West as a spinal manipulation, and is usually performed on the thoracic spine in order to mobilise individual vertebra that may be locked, causing restricted mobility in bending and rotating the spine.

An Ya Fu Wei Fa is considered to be a very Yang technique and, if performed incorrectly with too much force, can cause damage to the patient's spine and supporting ligaments. It is a form of passive joint manipulation, and should be performed only after all cautions and contraindications detailed within the Ban Fa technique (see page 195) have been ruled out.

- To perform An Ya Fu Wei Fa, ask the patient to lie face down in the prone position and stand to the patient's side.

- Place the palms of your hands on the patient's back at the level that you wish to manipulate, with the palm root of one hand over the transverse processes to the far side of the spine, and the minor thenar eminence of your other hand over the transverse processes to the near side of the spine. *Do not press directly on to the spine.*

- Stand with your body over your hands, as if performing chest compressions in first aid, and ask the patient to take a deep breath in. Then, as the patient breathes out, sink your weight through your hands and into their body.

- If necessary, apply Cun Jin (discussed later in the section of Ban Fa, on page 195) to the end of the movement just as the patient reaches full exhalation.

擦法 Ca Fa (to-and-fro rubbing)

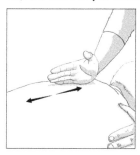
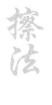
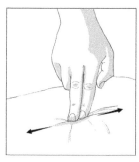
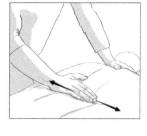

Technique category
Rubbing

Stages of treatment
Treatment stage, closing stage

Therapeutic actions
Ca Fa generates heat in order to activate the Jing Luo and promote the circulation of Qi and Blood. It warms the channels and local muscles, and can also be used to warm specific Zang Fu organs such as the Kidneys (when performed in the lumbar region) and the Stomach, Intestines and Uterus (when performed on the abdomen).

Ca Fa is a manipulation from the rubbing category that causes a great amount of heat, very quickly, as a result of friction. The technique can be used to generate heat at a superficial level, that can then also penetrate to the deeper levels of the channel system. Ca Fa is commonly used to cause expansion of the vessels and channels within the area in order to regulate the flow of Qi, bring warmth and nourishment into a specific area, resolve and disperse stagnation, and to treat Damp Cold Bi (痹) syndrome.

Due to the fact that Ca Fa can create such great amounts of heat within an area, it is never performed directly on to skin – Ca Fa would always require the use of oils, lotions or should be performed over clothing or a Tui Na blanket. In regards to oils and lotions, Ca Fa would commonly be used with oils or lotions such as Wood Lock Oil (see table on page 45) that enhances the warming and channel opening effects.

Method

Ca Fa can be performed with different parts of the hand depending on the area of the body being worked on, and depending on the desired amount of heat to be generated.

- With two fingers (very mild), the palm of the hand (mild), the major thenar eminence (moderate) or the minor thenar eminence (intense), rub to and fro in a linear direction along the channel or across a specific body area, approximately 100–120 times per minute.

- The force should be gentle to not move the skin, yet strong enough to generate heat. The distance should be as large as possible, and enough to cover beyond the injured site.

Tips

- The distance of travel for Ca Fa should be larger than the area of stagnation, as if to spread the Qi further afield and to improve circulation.

- Use different parts of the hand to increase or decrease the amount of heat produced (fingers, palm, major thenar eminence or minor thenar eminence).

- Pressure should be strong enough to produce heat, but light enough to prevent movement of the skin and body tissues.

Ca Fa must not be done directly onto skin as friction will cause too much heat and damage the skin. Ca Fa must be done over clothing/blanket or with oils/lotion.

搓法 Cuo Fa (palm twisting)

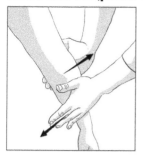
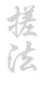

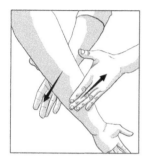
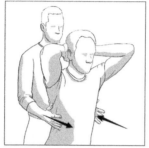

Technique category
Rubbing

Stages of treatment
Treatment stage, closing stage

Therapeutic actions
Cuo Fa helps to activate the Qi and Blood flow by separating the layers of tissue and unblocking the channels. It also does this by creating warmth within the channels and by opening the Qi Men.

Like Nian (捻), Cuo (搓) also means to twist, and in Tui Na particularly, it means to twist using the palms of the hand. It is a manipulation in which the practitioner uses the palms of the hand to twist and knead the major muscles and tissues of the limbs as well as the torso. It is particularly useful for dredging the channels and activating the flow of Qi and Blood by loosening the channels and separating the layers of tissue.

Method

Cuo Fa can be performed on any part of the body, although it is mostly used on the major muscle bellies of the limbs and on the torso. The speed is generally moderate to fast, although it can also be performed very slowly and gently whilst being combined with Na Fa, emphasising a stretching of the tissues at the same time.

- With the palms of the hands facing each other whilst holding a certain part of the body, apply inward pressure and rub the hands in opposite directions. The movement should be similar to making fire using sticks.

- Move the hands down, towards the extremities. Although the twisting movement should be quick, the downward movement of the hands should be relatively slow.

Tip

- Cuo Fa can also be used slowly on joints such as the shoulder or knees, for patients with cold conditions such as osteoarthritis. This would be performed for longer periods of time to generate Heat from the palms, and remain at the shoulder joint rather than moving down the limb. The speed would be slow enough to see very little movement.

抖法 **Dou Fa (shaking)**

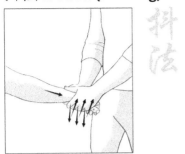

Technique category
Rubbing

Stages of treatment
Closing stage

Therapeutic actions
Dou Fa is used to remove obstructions from within the channels and joints (Qi Men) by essentially shaking them free, which helps to increase the flow of Qi and Blood throughout the limbs.

Dou (抖) means to shake, and refers to the shaking of the limbs to help shake free any obstruction within the channels and to open up the joints (Qi Men), therefore helping to increase the range of movement. It is most often used towards the end of treatment to help encourage the flow of Qi and Blood, and to relax the patient.

Method

Dou Fa is a simple technique that can be performed at moderate to high speeds with small amplitude. Slow shaking with large amplitude should be avoided as this may put too much force through the joints, causing damage to the ligaments.

- Take hold of the distal end of the patient's arm or leg with one or both hands, and make continuous up-and-down shaking movements of a small amplitude.

- Whilst holding the limb, lean back slightly to gain traction whilst shaking. This helps to greater relieve stagnation from within the joints.

- It is important to support the smaller joints such as the wrist and ankle, to prevent excessive force going through these joints. The lower limbs should also be shaken slightly slower and les vigorously than the upper limbs, due to their weight.

Tips

- The practitioner's arms must be relaxed and free, as to not exert force back into the neck or spine. The more relaxed the practitioner is, the more relaxed the patient will be.

- Try to create small wave-like movements travelling up the limb.

- Gentle traction to the joint will help to greater relieve stagnation from within the Qi Men.

滚法 **Gun Fa** (rolling)

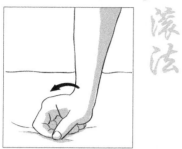

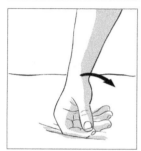

Technique category
Swaying

Stages of treatment
Opening stage, treatment stage

Therapeutic actions
Gun Fa is one of the most versatile techniques used within Tui Na, providing stimulation that can range anywhere between very light or very heavy. It promotes circulation, moves Blood stasis and activates the circulation of Qi throughout the channels. It also helps to relax tendons and relieve muscle spasms by warming and loosening the tissues. Gun Fa is particularly good for treating aching pain that is caused by Wind and Dampness, and is also widely used for neurological conditions such as neuralgia or numbness.

In relation to the other techniques that are used within Tui Na, Gun Fa is a relatively modern technique and was only developed and introduced to Tui Na in relatively more recent times from the technique of Yi Zhi Chan Tui Fa. That said, however, it is now one of the most used techniques within most styles of Tui Na, and is certainly one of the most recognisable. Gun Fa is also one of the few techniques that is unique to Tui Na. Most techniques that are used within Tui Na are used within many other styles of massage, such as Shiatsu or Western Sports Massage. Gun Fa, however, is used only in Tui Na with very specific principles behind the movement and technique.

Gun Fa is a useful technique to use during the treatment as it is very good to use both as an opening stage technique or during the treatment stage. When performed correctly, it is very easy to transfer a lot of power through the technique into the patient. For this reason, Gun Fa is commonly used when the patient has a strong constitution or is well covered either by muscle or adipose tissue. I would often hear it joked about amongst the Chinese Tui Na doctors that it is a technique used to treat the 'heavier' Western build.

Method

Gun Fa is a technique that has many variations depending on the area you are treating, the constitution and build of the patient and the desired therapeutic outcome. The main variation of Gun Fa is outlined here, with the most common variations detailed below.

- Use the phalangeal joints of the ring and little finger to make contact and 'roll' on a certain part of the body using the complex movement of extension/flexion of the wrist, along with swaying and minimal rotation of the forearm. The knuckle of the little finger should not break contact with the body.

- As the hand rolls to and fro, apply around three times more pressure to the forward roll than the backward roll, keeping contact the whole time. It is important to keep in contact with the body of the patient and not lift the hand off during the backward roll. The movement should have similar principles to using a rolling pin when rolling out dough. You do not lift the rolling pin, yet the roll forward is stronger than the roll back.

- The technique should be performed a comfortable 120–150 times per minute. This is not as fast as it sounds, and it is common to speed the technique up, causing an unsettled feeling to the patient. The rhythm and tempo of Gun Fa is important in order to create a hypnotic effect, which generates a calming sensation for the Shen.

- The power of the technique comes from the swing of the forearm that is generated from the shoulder rather than pressing forcefully down into the patient. The shoulders should be dropped and relaxed, and the arm should be held away from the body with the ability to fit a fist between the upper arm and the upper torso, and the elbow should be bent at around 120 degrees. It is important to not cross the body when performing Gun Fa as this will close off the shoulders and limit the amount of power that is able to be generated by the swing movement of the arm.

Precautions when using Gun Fa

- A common mistake of Gun Fa is to over-extend the wrist joint. This causes a misdirection of pressure through the wrist joint that can cause joint problems and damage to the extensor tendons if done over prolonged periods of time. Power comes from structure, and ensuring that the bones of the forearm and wrist are aligned helps to enable transfer of power safely into the patient.

- Another common mistake of Gun Fa is for the wrist to bend in an ulna/radial deviation rather than through the plane of extension and flexion (see the diagram below). This will put incorrect pressure on the carpal bones when applying any power through the technique, in particular, the scaphoid, hamate and pisiform bones, and cause injury to the ligaments within the wrist and can cause a radial or ulna impingement.

- It is important not to rub/scuff to avoid damage to the skin. Travelling with this technique should be done smoothly and very slowly, and should not be noticed by the patient. Gun Fa should never be done directly onto the skin, even with the use of oils. This is to protect the skin of both the practitioner and patient.

- It is important to gradually build power and strength over time whilst performing Gun Fa. Even though it may feel like you can apply a large amount of pressure relatively early on in the training of Gun Fa, unless the technique and hand positioning are correct, injury to the tendons of both the wrist and elbow can develop due to incorrect alignment.

Tips

- Movement should be 120–150 times per minute.

- Pressure should alternate from heavy (forward) to light (backward), being three times stronger forward than back.

- The shoulder and arm should be dropped and relax, and the elbow bends at an angle of 120 degrees.

Variations

With the following variations of Gun Fa, all of the principles that are applied to the standard method of Gun Fa should be applied here, unless otherwise stated.

四指滚法 Si Zhi Gun Fa

Performed straight, rolling from all four proximal interphalangeal joints of the fingers onto the phalangeal joints in a simple extension/flexion movement

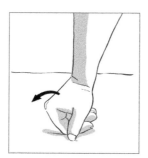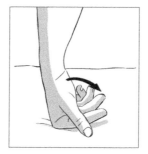

小魚際滾法 Xiao Yu Ji Gun Fa

Xiao Yu Ji refers to the minor thenar eminence (small fish belly), and is a variation of Gun Fa for use over weaker areas and bony areas, using the minor thenar eminence rather than phalangeal joints. This variation of Gun Fa is performed at a more oblique angle, with the pressure not as deep and the power not as strong due to the angle that it is performed at. Due to its oblique angle, this version is often called Xie Gun Fa, meaning oblique Gun Fa.

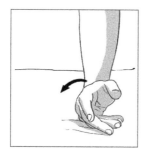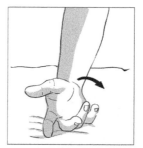

前臂滚法 Qian Bi Gun Fa

Qian Bi is the Chinese term for the forearm. Classically this area of the arm was known as the Dragon's Tail. By Using the forearm, much more pressure can be transferred into the patient and is a good variation to use when treating patients who have a very strong constitution or on areas that are very muscly. It is important that the movement of the forearm is in a linear direction, with pressure on the forward roll being around three times stronger than the backward roll.

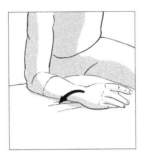 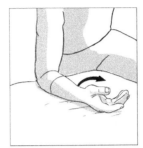

击法 Ji Fa (striking/percussing)

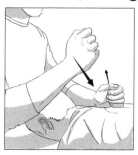

Technique category
Striking

Stages of treatment
Closing stage

Therapeutic actions
Ji Fa helps to increase the Blood flow and regulate the flow of Qi by dispersing stagnation. It works on the deeper layers of the body, and can also dislodge stagnations and obstructions from within the organs.

Ji (击) means to hit or to strike, and refers to the method of striking the surface of the body with a loose fist or the sides of the hand in a 'chopping' movement. It may also be called 'percussing'.

Much like Pai Fa, Ji Fa is one of the few techniques from the striking category, and is used during the treatment stage to disperse Qi and Blood, and during the closing stage to help disperse any stagnation that may have been caused by the treatment itself and to help bring the patient round to a more conscious state. Although similar to Pai Fa in that it is from the striking category, Ji Fa disperses Qi at a deeper level, whereas Pai Fa disperses Qi more superficially. This can be both felt and heard when using each technique. Ji Fa is also a technique that is also used momentarily for just one or two repetitions between certain techniques, such as Gun Fa, to assist in breaking up any stagnation in the area.

Method

When performing Ji Fa, it is important that the arms are kept relaxed so that force is transferred into the patient without rebounding back. Ji Fa can be done by one or both hands, and performed fast or slow in a drumming pattern. Rhythm is important for patient comfort.

- Make a loose fist (called a 'Sun Fist' due to being able to see light by looking through it), or have relaxed open palms.

- Strike the affected area steadily and rhythmically, approximately 120–240 times per minute, with the ulna side of the fist or open palm.

- This technique should *not* be performed over bone or over the vertebrae.

Tips

- The force of contact should build gradually, with excessive force being avoided.

- Shoulders and arms should be relaxed, and movement should come from pivoting at the elbow.

- Ji Fa is good in cases of respiratory conditions, and can be used to help dislodge phlegm that is stuck in the chest.

摇法 Ma Fa (wiping)

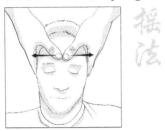

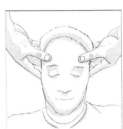

Technique category
Rubbing

Stages of treatment
Opening stage, treatment stage

Therapeutic actions
Ma Fa generates a gentle warmth within the more superficial channels, and can help to relax tension within the smaller muscles groups. Ma Fa also helps to calm the Shen due to its gentle and soft nature.

Ma (摇) means to wipe, and is often used on parts of the body that are more sensitive due to a greater amount of nerve endings, such as the face and the sternum, and areas that are more bony. It is a simple technique, and has a very calming affect due to its soft and gentle movements.

Method

Ma Fa should be done very lightly and superficially using the pads of the thumbs, although it should be strong enough to affect the Sinew channels rather than just the skin. It is most commonly performed with two thumbs symmetrically, although one thumb can also be used. Ma Fa is often used on the face and hands to help relieve tension and to calm the mind.

- Place the whole pad of the thumb on to a part of the body, such as the forehead, and wipe across the surface of the skin.

- The fingers should be completely relaxed, resting on the patient if necessary.

- The thumbs should not lose contact and have a continuous and smooth movement.

- Direction of the wipe should be one way, rather than backwards and forwards.

Tips

- Although Ma Fa should not be performed too strongly, as this would then become Tui Fa, it should also not be too light, as we want to affect the Sinew channels and not just the skin regions.

- Ma Fa is often used with lubrication, especially if the skin is dry.

- Try applying Rou Fa with the thumb on Yin Tang followed by an arching Ma Fa movement from Yin Tang to Tai Yang, followed by Rou Fa again on Tai Yang.

摩法 Mo Fa (circular rubbing)

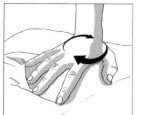

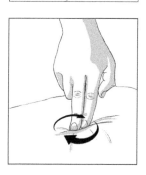

Technique category
Rubbing

Stages of treatment
Opening stage, treatment stage

Therapeutic actions
Mo Fa provides light and moderate stimulations to the superficial layers of the body to stimulate the Wei Qi within the cutaneous regions and the Sinew channels. By creating warmth to the area and stimulating the Wei Qi, Mo Fa also helps to regulate the flow of Qi and Blood to soothe pain and relax the Sinew channels. Due to its gentle, rhythmical and warming action, Mo Fa can also be used to help calm the Shen.

Mo Fa is a technique from the 'rubbing' category, and is one of the oldest techniques that originated from the more 'instinctual' methods of primitive bodywork. It is performed in a circular motion with either the palm or the fingers, and is a very simple technique that can be used for a number of reasons. Its main use is to warm and nourish the tissues. By warming the body tissues, it can help to open the channels and promote the circulation of Qi and Blood. Mo Fa is also used to introduce physical contact to the patient at the beginning of treatment. The technique enables the patient to relax and feel comfortable with physical touch before heavier or more stimulating techniques are used.

Another reason to use Mo Fa is to allow practitioners to feel the contours of the body and to feel for any excesses or deficiencies, abnormalities or tensions within the body among other things. It can essentially be used as a type of palpation diagnosis. When performing Mo Fa, it is important to ensure that the fingers are completely relaxed and to move with the contours of the patient's body, enabling the practitioner to feel what is happening underneath the hand without any tension interfering with the senses.

Mo Fa is performed very superficially, without the body tissues moving underneath. There is little pressure applied to the technique, with pressure coming from relaxation and the weight of the hand, and applied uniformly through the whole hand.

Method

When performing Mo Fa, it is important to keep the hand and wrist completely relaxed, allowing movement to come from the arm, and allowing the movements to feel consistent and rhythmical – much like a mop being controlled and led by its handle.

- Fix the whole palm surface or the pads of the fingers on to a certain part of the body, and make gentle rhythmic circular movements with the wrist and forearm together.

- When performing Mo Fa with the palm of the hand, the intent should be focused on P-8 (Lao Gong).

- Pressure should be light, yet confident, with little force, and circular movements should be performed at around 120 times per minute.

- The direction of the circular movements should be led by the radial aspect of the arm when moving towards your body, then led by the ulna aspect of the arm when moving away from your body.

- There should not be any tension in the wrist joint, enabling free movement and complete relaxation of the hand.

Tips

- This technique can be used both diagnostically and therapeutically.

- Mo Fa also stimulates the cutaneous channels and promotes stimulation of the Wei Qi.

- The wrist and hand should be completely relaxed, allowing gentle rhythmical movements that are led by the arm.

- Pressure should be firm and confident, whilst *not* moving the tissues beneath the hand.

拿法 Na Fa (grasping)

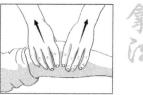

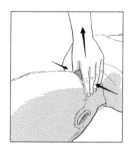

Technique category
Pressing

Stages of treatment
Treatment stage

Therapeutic actions
Na Fa breaks down scar tissue and can also be used to reduce spasm by relaxing the tendons. It helps to move Blood and stops pain, and is good for discharging tension from the larger muscle groups by separating the fibres.

Na Fa is considered to be one of the core techniques used within Tui Na, and its importance is reflected in the fact that it is included in the name of the therapy, Tui Na. Na (拿) literally means to grasp, or to take hold of, and the technique has its roots in the Chinese Martial Arts application of Qin Na (擒拿). Within Tui Na, Na Fa refers to grasping of the muscles or body tissues, and pulling them away from their original position, in addition to energetically taking away from the body. Na Fa can be used almost anywhere on the body, although the technique is used mainly on the looser muscle groups that can be pulled away from their original position, such as the nape of the neck, the shoulders, arms and the leg muscles.

Method

- Using the pads of the thumb with the index and middle finger, or all four fingers to grasp certain parts of the body (such as large muscle bellies), pull the muscle away from the body and release.
- Repeat this technique in a rhythmical pattern.
- Exertion of force may be from light to heavy, although sudden heavy exertion should be avoided, as this can cause the patient to tense up in defence.
- Avoid using the tips of the fingers or thumb to ensure that you are not digging the fingers into the patient. Avoid pinching.

Tips

- Once the tissue has been grasped away from the bone, it can be shaken slightly to further move Qi and Blood, and reduce stagnation.

- The practitioner can introduce a complex movement, by kneading the tissues at the same time as grasping and releasing. This is sometimes referred to as 'grasping with internal rubbing'.

捻法 Nian Fa (finger twisting)

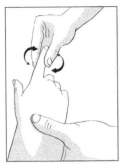

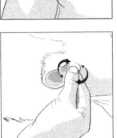

Technique category
Rubbing

Stages of treatment
Treatment stage, closing stage

Therapeutic actions
Nian Fa activates the Qi and Blood flow by causing stimulation along a channel in addition to warming and unblocking the channels. It helps to mobilise and lubricate the joints whilst creating space within the Qi Men, and can also stimulate acupoints.

Nian (捻) means to twist, and particularly means to twist using the fingers. It is a manipulation in which the practitioner uses the fingers (usually the index finger and thumb) to rub and knead small joints, tendons, small muscle bellies and the ears. It is particularly useful at the extremities for releasing the Sinew channels and stimulating the Jing Well points, and treating stiffness of the smaller joints.

Method

Nian Fa can be performed on any part of the body, although it is mostly used on the fingers, toes, ears, any small joint or small muscle belly and along specific channels.

- With the pads of the index finger and thumb, take hold of the patient's affected area and hold each side, as if pinching the joint. Apply opposite pressure with the finger and thumb towards each other, and gently twist backwards and forwards whilst also kneading.

- The movement should be similar to rolling a small piece of clay between the finger and thumb.

Tips

- Nian Fa can be used effectively on specific Acupuncture points on the hands and feet.

- When performing on the fingers or toes, it is sometimes helpful to use small amounts of lubrication, such as An Mo Rou.

捏法 Nie Fa (pinching)

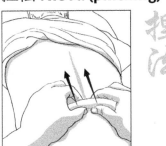

Technique category
Pressing

Stages of treatment
Treatment stage

Therapeutic actions
By lifting the tissues away from the body, Nie Fa allows the free circulation of Qi and Blood in areas that are usually tight and stagnant, such as the flesh that covers the spine. Nie Fa is commonly used to regulate the circulation surrounding the Spine.

Nie Fa is mainly a technique used within paediatric Tui Na (Xiao Er Tui Na), although it is also useful on adults, especially to help regulate the nervous system through regulating the Qi and Blood flow along the Du channel.

Method

Nie Fa is often done along the Du channel and inner Bladder channel in adults, but can be done on any fleshy part of body.

- Pinch the body tissue between the thumbs and the first two (or three) fingers.

- The force exerted between the fingers and thumb should be even and soft, with the force being just enough to hold the flesh away from the body.

- The practitioner can then 'walk' their fingers along the body, keeping the tissue pinched between the thumbs and fingers. It is important to avoid any twisting or rotating.

- It is important that the pads of the thumbs and fingers be used rather than the tips.

拍法 Pai Fa (patting)

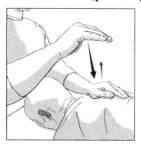

Technique category
Striking

Stages of treatment
Treatment stage, closing stage

Therapeutic actions
Pai Fa strongly moves and invigorates the Qi and Blood at the superficial layers of the body by stimulating the Wei Qi. Due to its action at the superficial layers of the body, it is excellent at releasing exterior Wind from the channels and bringing pathogens to the exterior (especially when performed on the upper back).

Pai (拍) means to pat, and refers to the method of patting the surface of the body with an empty, or hollow, hand. Pai Fa is one of the few techniques from the striking category of techniques, and is used during treatment to disperse Qi and Blood, and at the end of treatment to help disperse any stagnation that may have been caused by the treatment itself.

Classically, Pai Fa was used to remove Wind from the channels, due to its superficial dispersing nature. It is similar to Ji Fa, in that it disperses Qi through a striking movement; however, Pai Fa disperses Qi at the superficial level, whereas Ji Fa disperses Qi at deeper levels. This can be both felt and heard when using each technique.

Method

When performing Pai Fa, it is important to keep an 'empty palm' to avoid causing a 'slap' sensation that could cause discomfort to the patient. Pai Fa can be done by one or two hands, and performed fast or slow.

- Make a hollow in the palm of the hand by gently squeezing the sides of the fingers and thumb together, and slightly flexing the metacarpophalangeal joints. Once a 'cupping' shape has been made with the hands, the movement should be led by the wrist and elbows, with the hands completely relaxed.

- Pat the affected area steadily and rhythmically, approximately 120 times per minute.

- The centre of the palm should *not* come into contact with the body, creating a pocket of air when the rest of the hand makes contact.

- The technique should not be done for too long, or if the skin develops redness, as this can have the opposite effect.

Tips

- When performing Pai Fa, it is important to keep the shoulders down, with the elbows and wrists relaxed so that the vibration caused does not travel back up the arms, into the neck, and create discomfort.

- This manipulation is good for performing on the upper back in cases of respiratory conditions in order to disperse phlegm and expel Wind.

揉法 Rou Fa (kneading)

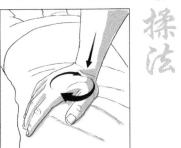

Technique category
Swaying

Stages of treatment
Opening stage, treatment stage

Therapeutic actions
Rou Fa is a versatile technique, providing both light and heavy stimulation that affects the Qi and Blood at the superficial and deep layers respectively. It can be used to help promote the circulation of Qi and Blood and warms the channels, in addition to calming the Shen due to its warming and relaxing movement. It may also be used to stimulate specific acupuncture points when performed with the thumb.

Almost like a combination of Mo Fa and An Fa, this manipulation uses the technique and movement of Mo Fa, with the pressure of An Fa. Unlike Mo Fa, however, Rou Fa is more static on the surface, and instead moves the tissues underneath the skin. In addition to the palm, the forearm (Qian Bi) or thumb (Mu Zhi) may also be used for larger or more specific areas respectively.

Rou Fa is one of the most commonly used techniques in many modalities of bodywork, and like Gun Fa, it is a useful technique to use during the treatment as it is good to use both as an opening stage technique or during the treatment stage due to its versatility in pressure and speed. When performed correctly, it is easy to transfer much power through the technique into the patient, whether using the palm root, fingers or even the forearm.

Method

Rou Fa can be performed with different parts of the hand and arm, depending on the area of the body being worked on and depending on the amount of pressure needed. The following explains how to perform Rou Fa using the palm root.

- Place the palm root on to a part of the body, and make gentle circular movements with enough pressure to move the tissues beneath the surface of the body.

- The speed should be around 120 times per minute.

- The hand should move the deeper tissues rather than rubbing the surface, to allow the warmth generated at the palm root to penetrate deeply into the body.

- Movement should be generated from the swaying movement of the arm, and strength should be generated from posture and structure, with minimal use of the muscles.

Tips

- The power of this technique comes from the swinging motion of the arm.

- The arm should be relaxed, and power transferred from the trunk of the body.

- Pressure should not be too strong, and the patient should feel comfortable.

- The tempo and rhythm of Rou Fa should be similar to Gun Fa, and the two can be interchanged at various stages of treatment.

Variations
大魚際揉法 Da Yu Ji Rou Fa

This technique looks and feels quite different to the other variations of Rou Fa, and makes use of the major thenar eminence (Da Yu Ji). This variation should be done much quicker with slightly less pressure. This is ideal for headaches and facial pain when used on the head, as it can relax the soft tissues that cover the skull without requiring much perpendicular pressure. Movement should be rapid and relaxed, as if waving quickly or attempting to shake water off the fingers.

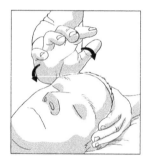

前臂揉法 Qian Bi Rou Fa

Qian Bi Rou Fa, meaning 'kneading with the forearm' (Qian Bi), is useful when needing to get deep into stronger areas. It is also useful when the practitioner is feeling tired, as power can be transferred through the forearm very easily using the body structure. It is most often used on the hamstrings and back in the prone position, or on the shoulders and side of the neck in the seated position. It is important that, when performing Rou Fa with the forearm, the wrist and hand are completely relaxed and 'switched off'.

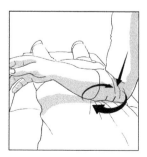

拇指揉法 Mu Zhi Rou Fa

Mu Zhi Rou Fa, meaning 'kneading with the thumb' (Mu Zhi), is used when needing to perform Rou Fa on specific points, such as Acupuncture points or Ashi points. Pressure is applied perpendicularly through the pad of the thumb, with small circular movements to stimulate the point.

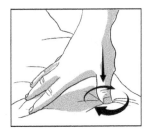

弹拨法 Tan Bo Fa (plucking)

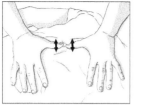

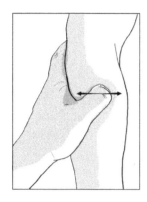

Technique category
Pressing

Stages of treatment
Treatment stage

Therapeutic actions
Tan Bo Fa is most commonly used to break down scar tissue and to separate adhesions found within the Sinew channels. It can also be used to stop pain and relax the Sinew channels by encouraging the movement of Qi and Blood to resolving Qi stagnation and Blood stasis and facilitate localised healing. Tan Bo Fa is also used to develop strength and flexibility in the tendons, which is particularly useful for treating injuries and joint weakness in the elderly.

Tan Bo Fa means to pluck, and specifically, it means to pluck an instrument string (as opposed to plucking feathers) as it is performed by plucking over tendons, sinews or taut muscle fibres in order to cause relaxation of the tissues. It is considered to be a strong 'Yang'-style technique, and is commonly used to break down scar tissue and separate adhesions, which can be quite uncomfortable for the patient due to the powerful nature of the technique. For this reason, it is important that Tan Bo Fa is only used during the treatment stage once the Sinew channels have been sufficiently opened, warmed and relaxed. What's more, due to the Yang nature of Tan Bo Fa, when the technique is performed powerfully it should only be used for short periods at a time (no longer than 30 seconds), with dispersing techniques used in between.

Tan Bo Fa can also be used (in a milder fashion) to gently break down the sinews and tendons in order to encourage a greater flow of Qi and Blood to the area. This enables the sinews and tendons to develop more strength. In China, Tan Bo Fa technique is used in this way on the elderly so that the connective tissues tighten up and give more stability to the joints, as sinew and tendon strength is considered to be more important in old age. An example of this would be to apply Tan Bo Fa to the major tendons of the knees, in order to allow greater stability and flexibility of the knees.

Method

Tan Bo Fa is a relatively straightforward technique in application; however, extreme care must be taken due to its potentially harsh and damaging nature.

- Exert pressure with the tip of the thumb or the radial side of the thumb perpendicularly against a tendon or muscle.

- Pluck across the muscles fibres back and forth, like playing a stringed instrument. The four fingers should be relaxed and placed statically on the local area or gently rub across the surface of the skin only for support of the thumb.

- The force of the technique should increase gradually, to minimise discomfort to the patient.

- When performing Tan Bo Fa, the thumb should be working directly on the sinews and moving the muscle fibres rather than merely rubbing and creating friction on the surface of the skin.

- If the technique requires more strength than is comfortable when using just one thumb, two thumbs can be overlapped, or the palm root of the non-dominant hand can be placed over the thumb performing the technique.

- Techniques such as Mo Fa, Ca Fa or light Rou Fa should be used immediately after Tan Bo Fa to help reduce any stagnation that has potentially been caused by the strong nature of Tan Bo Fa.

Tips

- Tan Bo Fa is a very 'Yang' technique, and should be done only when the Sinew channels have been opened and warmed.

- Use dispersing techniques frequently when performing Tan Bo Fa strongly in order to help reduce stagnation and discomfort.

- When performing Tan Bo Fa with the thumb on areas with lots of tension (such as the back), two thumbs may be overlapped for increased strength, or the palm root of the non-dominant hand can be placed over the thumb performing the technique, with pressure being applied through the palm rather than relying on the strength of the thumb.

推法 Tui Fa (pushing)

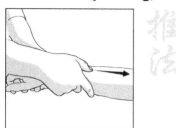

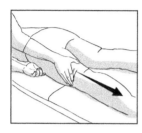

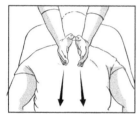

Technique category
Rubbing

Stages of treatment
Opening stage, treatment stage, closing stage

Therapeutic actions
Tui Fa is one of the most versatile techniques used within Tui Na, and can be used during any stage of treatment as it can be performed both powerfully and softly. Depending on the variation, it may be used to dredge the channels, help to move Qi and Blood and calm the Shen by causing relaxation. It may also be used to warm the Sinew channels and, when performed more forcefully, be used to break down tension and stagnation within the tissues.

Tui Fa means to push, and is used to push along parts of the body in a single line. The technique may consist of finger pushing, palm pushing, elbow pushing or other parts of the body, and is a single directional movement that should be done rhythmically as quickly as 120–150 times per minute.

Method

Tui Fa is a technique that allows us to adapt in many ways depending on the patient's body type, presenting condition, desired effect or even practitioner preference. Tui Fa can be performed with the thumb, various parts of the hand, forearm or the elbow, and can be used softly or powerfully. The three most common methods of Tui Fa are described below:

Using the thumb to Tui (推) *along* the Sinew channels

- Place the pad of the thumb on to the body, and push in a straight line along the direction of the Sinew channel (the direction should be lined up with the metacarpal of the thumb).

- Once the thumb has made contact with the body and is positioned correctly, the forearm and hand should be completely relaxed whilst maintaining structure.

- Movement should come from the extension of the elbow in a forward direction.

- This method can be replicated with the fingers, minor thenar eminence, palm root or elbow.

Using the thumb to Tui (推) *across* the Sinew channels

- Place the thumb on to the body, perpendicular to the direction of the channel, and rest the fingers in a relaxed fan shape, with the thumb in line with the direction of movement.

- Use the fingers as a pivot (without losing contact), and move the forearm in a way that the wrist flexes and extends whilst the thumb moves across the tissues.

- Movement should come from the sway of the forearm from the shoulder, much like Gun Fa.

Using the 'Tiger's Mouth' (虎口, Hu Kou) to dredge the channels

The 'Tiger's Mouth' refers to the arch of the hand formed with the hand stretched open by the first finger and thumb (used to grip around something). It is primarily used to dredge the channels, and is used along the limbs moving outwards towards the extremities.

- With the 'Tiger's Mouth', place the hand on to the body, and push along a channel in a straight line.

- Pressure should be slow and firm, and movement continuous in order to dredge the channel (imagine squeezing paste out of a tube).

Tips

- The power of this technique again comes from the swinging of the forearm, not from the wrist or the finger/thumb joints.

- Pressure should be steady and even. When using the palm to 'dredge' the channels, pushing should be slow and firm.

- To-and-fro rubbing should be avoided – this is an entirely different technique. Force should be exerted in one direction, to 'push' the tissues.

- Lotions, oils or balms may be used on certain areas of the body.

Variations
推法 Fen Tui Fa

Fen means to separate, with Fen Tui Fa meaning to use Tui Fa in two opposite directions – also known as 'separating Yin and Yang'. This technique is where two hands are used, and the thumbs push in two opposite directions. It is most commonly used on the palms of the hands and on the back.

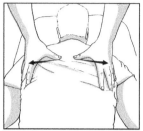
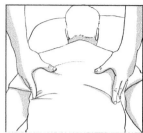

推法 Gui Tui Fa

Gui means to 'kneel'. Using the interphalangeal joint of the thumb (with the thumb bent, as if it's 'kneeling' down), this technique puts more concentrated force on to a specific area, and has a little less movement due to the structure of the thumb. It is used in the same way that the elbow might be used in order to exert more force on to a concentrated area. Gui Tui Fa is often used on the palm of the hand to access the spaces between the metacarpals, and also at the nape of the neck on points such as GB-20 (Feng Chi), BL-10 (Tian Zhu) and DU-16 (Feng Fu).

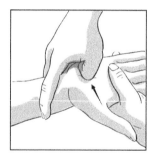

推法 Si Zhi Tui Fa

In this variation, the first three fingers are in contact with the patient in addition to the thumb, and are also utilised in the pushing movement (rather than being used for stability). The majority of the focus is still, however, on the thumb, with the fingers just gently rubbing on the patient in the surrounding areas for an analgesic and desensitising affect, which can be useful when performing on areas that are sensitive or painful.

振法 Zhen Fa (vibrating)

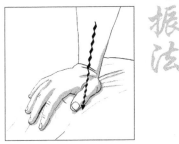

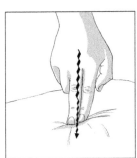

Technique category
Vibrating

Stages of treatment
Treatment stage

Therapeutic actions
Zhen Fa is a relatively gentle technique in regards to physical pressure, but can be incredibly powerful energetically, to help move Blood and remove obstruction from deep within the body. It helps to calm the mind and can strongly warm the area, which also results in relaxation of the tissues.

Zhen Fa, meaning 'vibrating technique', is actually a form of Wai Qi Liao Fa, which is essentially Qi emission and should in no way be tension of the tissues. Due to the nature of the Nei Gong training needed to perform this technique correctly as it was intended, it is a difficult technique, and something I am yet unable to do properly myself – it takes many years of training in Nei Gong in order to perform what may be considered as Qi emission strong enough to be used in the way that Zhen Fa is indicated.

Zhen Fa is indeed commonly used by many practitioners with little or no training in Qi Gong or Nei Gong; however, this is a very mechanical way of doing the technique, and has a different effect that cannot penetrate as deeply (which is not the same as the technique that was developed hundreds of years ago). Even expansion of the Yi (intent) is not enough to perform Zhen Fa properly. Due to the actual complex nature of the traditional technique of Zhen Fa, it isn't covered in this book as it is really just an end product of a much more in-depth technique involving Nei Gong that could be a whole book in itself. However, below I explain how to perform the modern approach to Zhen Fa, developed for modern practitioners with little or no internal arts training.

Method

To perform Zhen Fa, the practitioner should have their body as relaxed as possible, using only enough contraction to cause gentle vibration of the minor muscles of the arm.

- Place the hand, or the fingertips, on to the body and make very fast and very small vibrating movements with the whole arm. The movement should resemble a tremble.

- The vibrating movement should be of an up-and-down movement, and transferred into the patient's body, creating warmth and relaxation.

Tips

- The direction of the vibration should be up and down, perpendicular to the body, rather than side to side.

- This technique is excellent for breaking up and moving stagnations, such as constipation if done on the abdomen.

一指禅推法 Yi Zhi Chan Tui Fa (single finger meditation pushing)

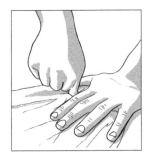

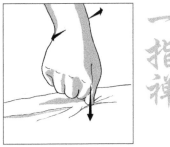

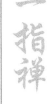

Technique category
Swaying

Stages of treatment
Treatment stage

Therapeutic actions
Yi Zhi Chan is essentially the Tui Na practitioner's acupuncture needle. Its main therapeutic action is to stimulate acupoints and activate the channels. It is able to relax the tendons and muscles due to its continual rhythmic movement, and helps to eliminate Qi and Blood stagnation in order to reduce pain. When used on areas such as the abdomen, it is also useful for dispersing accumulations such as food retention or constipation.

Yi Zhi Chan Tui (一指禅推) is commonly interpreted as single finger meditation pushing. However, Chan (禅) does not directly mean meditation, and like the Dao (道) of Daoism, it cannot really be explained in words. It is the Chinese pronunciation of the more common Japanese term Zen of Zen Buddhism, and is generally considered to mean a number of things that lead to the 'path to enlightenment'.

Yi Zhi Chan Tui Fa is essentially the Tui Na practitioner's needle. The technique is mainly used on acupuncture points or Ashi points for longer periods of time in order to activate and stimulate the point, and also used on areas of accumulation such as the abdomen in cases of food retention or constipation.

Yi Zhi Chan Tui Fa is a manipulation in which the thumb exerts pressure on to a single point, whilst performing a slight rocking action with the forearm and hand to add a vibrational stimulation to the point. It can be done anywhere on the body, and is performed at around 120–240 times per minute. The slower movements act on a deeper layer, and more force can be exerted, with the higher speed using less pressure and working along the more superficial layers of the body. The finger, hand and arm should be very relaxed, as this allows the technique to sink and expand into the patient's body, which can often give a sensation of De Qi.

Method

Despite how it looks, Yi Zhi Chan Tui Fa is a difficult technique to master, mainly due to the intent and direction of pressure. It is very easy to accidentally 'jump' or 'slide' off the point of contact, or for the pressure to dissipate at the surface of the body. If this happens, ensure that the weight of the arm is dropped and relaxed, and the mind is focused just below the point of contact.

- With your stance square on the patient, place the tip of the thumb on to the patient's body, either on an acupoint or an Ashi point, with the thumbnail facing towards your midline.

- Pull the fingers into the palm of the hand, as if to make a very loose fist, with the side of the index finger resting just above the first joint of the thumb. This helps to give the thumb some support.

- Gently sway the forearm so that the thumb joint rocks back and forth whilst at the same time applying pressure perpendicularly into the patient. The hand and arm should be completely relaxed, with the full dead weight being transferred through the tip of the thumb. It is important at this stage to focus the intent directly into the patient so that the vibration travels into the body rather than side to side, across the surface of the body.

- Rock the thumb back and forth around 120–240 times per minute, depending on the desired depth.

Tips

- The shoulder, wrist and elbow should be kept relaxed, but not lax.

- The weight of the arm should transfer through the thumb and into the patient.

- Ensure that the pressure is travelling perpendicularly into the body rather than dispersing at the surface.

- Yi Zhi Chan is essentially the Tui Na practitioner's needle in respect to stimulating acupuncture points.

PASSIVE JOINT MANIPULATION TECHNIQUES

The following three techniques are from within the passive joint manipulation category, and are a little more complex in nature than the previous techniques. This is largely due to the fact that care must be taken to keep all movements within natural anatomical ranges, and that they are both safe and comfortable to the patient. What's more, practitioner positioning and posture are extremely important for passive joint manipulation techniques. This is for both strength and again, safe practice. All techniques within this section should be performed within the treatment stage, once the channels have been suitably opened and warmed up.

拔伸法 Ba Shen Fa (traction)

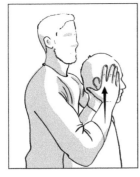
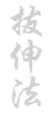

Technique category
Passive joint manipulation

Stages of treatment
Treatment stage

Therapeutic actions
Ba Shen Fa is used to help move Qi and Blood that may have become stagnated within the joints by essentially creating space. It is also used to reset and realign small joints, relieve joint pain and open up any joint compression.

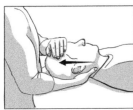
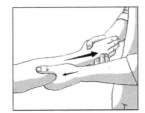

Ba (拔) means to pull, and Shen (伸) means to stretch, with Ba Shen being used to refer to the manoeuvre of traction. Traction from a Western medical perspective generally means to pull and extend in a neutral plain, and may be performed on almost any joint. However, when used in Tui Na, the movement is not *always* done along a neutral plane, and depends on the joint and desired outcome.

Ba Shen Fa is essentially performed by fixing one end of a joint or limb, and pulling and drawing the other end in order to open out the space within the joint. It is not necessary to create huge amounts of space, but just enough for any stagnation to be released and for the joint to become decompressed and mobile again. Although Ba Shen Fa can be done on any joint, it is most commonly done on the neck, back, hips, knee, ankle, shoulder, wrist and finger joints.

Within Chinese Medicine, Qi, Blood and Body Fluids flow in and out of the joints through what are known as the Qi Men (齐门, Qi gates). It is at these gates that the substances of the body are most likely to stagnate. Imagine a six-lane motorway bottlenecking to a two-lane motorway before expanding back again into a six-lane motorway. This is why most inflammation and long-term damage is likely to build up within the joints (such as arthritis and even eczema). Using Ba Shen Fa allows more space within the joint for the Qi and Body Fluids to flow more freely without obstruction, and also relieve any compression that may be hindering the flow of Qi, Blood and Body Fluids.

Note: This technique should not be done on weak joints, lax joints or recent dislocations/ subluxations. Ba Shen Fa can temporarily destabilise a joint.

Method

Depending on which joint is being manipulated, Ba Shen Fa is adapted slightly to work most efficiently with that particular joint. Most methods of Ba Shen Fa are performed in a neutral plane of movement, and require one part of the joint to be fixed whilst the other is pulled away. However, some joints (such as the knee) require more arching movements to enable a 'prising open' of the joint. Each time Ba Shen Fa is applied, it is a good idea to hold the stretch for around 30 seconds, or whatever is comfortable for the patient.

Once the stretch has been held for the desired time, it is important that the joint is released slowly whilst the patient is breathing out. Rapidly letting go of the stretch can cause sudden pain and discomfort within the joint, especially if the compression was painful in the first place.

Head/neck

Ba Shen Fa can be performed on the head and neck in either a seated position or a supine position. Both are beneficial, and ultimately depend on the practitioner's preference or treatment planning.

- **Seated:** With the patient sitting up, place your thumbs on either side of the head in the region of GB-20 (Feng Chi), and place the hands at the side of the head – create a V-shape with the thumb and index finger and avoid pressing into the ears. When the patient is comfortable and relaxed, lift the head slightly and gently directly upwards, and hold. It is best to keep your arms in a fixed position and lift using the legs. This avoids having to use arm leverage or strength.

- **Supine:** With the patient lying on their back, take hold of the occiput with one hand, and place the other hand on top of the patient's forehead. This is to keep the patient's head in a neutral plane and prevent it from tilting forwards. Pull the patient's head gently into a neutral plane and hold.

Shoulder

There are a wide number of ways that Ba Shen Fa can be used on the shoulder, depending on the nature of the injury or condition. The most important thing about performing Ba Shen Fa on the shoulder is that there is no laxity in the joint, and that the technique is performed in a neutral plane.

- For general traction of the shoulder, with the patient sitting up simply take hold of the patient's forearm with one hand, and place your other hand on top of their shoulder proximal to the shoulder joint to fix it in place. Pull the patient's arm in a neutral plane towards your hip (this helps to use your structure rather than raw strength). Hold the traction for a few seconds then release.

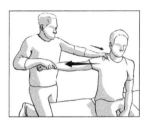

Back

Ba Shen Fa on the back can be difficult without a proper traction table as the patient is likely to slide before sufficient traction is created, and it is unhelpful for the patient to brace themselves by holding on to something. That said, gentle traction of the back (especially the lower back) can be very therapeutic.

- Ask the patient to lie on their back in a supine position, and take hold of both legs just above the ankles. Lift the legs slightly so that they are away from the treatment couch, and lean back using your body weight to create traction in the back. Hold this position.

Hip

Ba Shen Fa on the hip can be difficult only because there is generally a lot of strength within the tissues holding the hips in place, and there is also generally a lot of compression within the hips due to the nature of our upright posture.

- Ba Shen Fa on the hips is best performed with the patient lying on their back in a relaxed supine position. With the patient's legs straight, take hold of the patient's affected leg just above the ankle. This is to ensure that the ankle does not absorb any energy of the technique. Make sure that the patient's leg is not abducted greater that 30 degrees, and lean back whilst pulling on the leg in a neutral plane. Hold this position.

Knee

Performing Ba Shen Fa on the knee is slightly different to most other joints due to the fact that the knee is a hinge joint, and does not respond easily to traction along a neutral plane. What we need to do is to 'prise' open the joint using leverage.

- With the patient lying on their back in a relaxed supine position, ask the patient to bend their affected leg and put their foot flat on the treatment couch. Place your forearm directly behind the knee in the popliteal fossa, and lift the knee up slightly so that the patient's foot comes off the bed. With your other hand, take hold of the patient's leg just above the ankle, and push their heel backwards towards their thigh. With your forearm positioned behind the patient's knee, this should open up the knee joint.

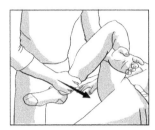

Ankle

Although it is important to check the stability of any joint before performing Ba Shen Fa, it is especially important when treating the ankle. This is mainly due to the simple fact that the ankle supports and transfers the weight of the whole body.

- With the patient lying in a relaxed supine position, take hold of the back of the patient's heel with one hand and place the other hand over the top of the foot. Pull the foot in a neutral plane away from the body.

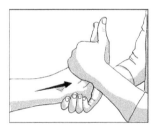

Tips

- It is most important to use your body weight, structure and proper leverage whilst performing Ba Shen Fa, and avoid using raw strength. This will protect both the practitioner and the patient.

- It is important to stay relaxed and comfortable when performing Ba Shen Fa, especially when performing on the neck.

- Be subtle with your movements, even when first taking hold of the patient. If you come across as threatening, even subconsciously, the patient's body will tighten due to an instinctual response, and the technique will be ineffective.

扳法 Ban Fa (pulling and/or twisting)

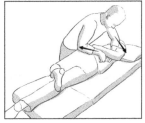

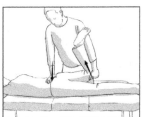

Technique category
Passive joint manipulation

Stages of treatment
End of the treatment stage

Ban Fa is a technique used to increase mobility to parts of the spine, and to realign tissues and misplaced joints, most commonly to the spine and the shoulder. Traditionally, Ban Fa was used as part of Zheng Gu (正骨), which was the practice of bone setting, and is primarily used to realign dislocated joints and displaced vertebrae as a result of trauma, similar to chiropractic and osteopathic manipulations.

Using Ban Fa encourages and allows the Qi and Blood to flow smoothly by reducing obstructions or stagnations of the free flow caused by joints sitting in unnatural positions. If joints are not sitting out of place, however, Ban Fa may still be used simply as an assisted stretch to increase the flow of Qi and Blood through the Jing Luo system by re-establishing the correct pathways and alignments of the muscles and tissues along the Jin Jing (Tendon/Sinew channels).

Cun Jin (寸勁)

Cun Jin, meaning 'short power', is essentially the equivalent to a Grade 5 manipulation or high velocity low amplitude thrust (also known as a HVT or HVLAT) that may be used in Osteopathy or Chiropractic practice.

When performing Ban Fa to adjust the skeletal structure, it is important that Cun Jin is applied. The overstretch that is used to adjust and manipulate the joints needs to be very quick in speed and very short in distance (almost like a twitch) in order to be effective and safe. Until you have the ability to apply Cun Jin effectively, Ban Fa is best used as an assisted stretch.

If performed correctly, there should be very little force needed with Ban Fa. Once the surrounding tissues and muscles have been warmed and relaxed sufficiently, causing the muscles and tissues to sit correctly, adjustments of the joints happen very easily and smoothly – this will produce far better results than a forced adjustment. My thoughts are, that if it has to be forced back into alignment, then it is not ready to go back (and is unlikely to stay there).

Safe practice

Ban Fa is an advanced technique, and comes with more cautions and contraindications than other Tui Na techniques. Care and concentration must be given.

Cautions and contraindications

In addition to the standard cautions and contraindications of Tui Na discussed in Section 1, Ban Fa carries its own due to the nature of the technique. Unless all cautions and contraindications have been established, you should not use Ban Fa. Although very safe if performed correctly and responsibly, Ban Fa has the most contraindications of any other Tui Na technique and should be performed with great care.

Cautions	
Bone and tissue disorders	Disk herniation and disk protrusion Inflammatory joint processes Hypermobility or ligamentous laxity Minor osteoporosis Iatrogenic (e.g. long treatment with steroids)
Vascular disorders	Arterial calcification Medicamentous anticoagulation Arterial hypertension
Other	Vertigo Pregnancy Systemic infections Psychological Growing children
Contraindications	
Bone and tissue disorders	Post-traumatic instability (e.g. dislocation, luxation, ruptured ligaments) Osteoporosis Tumours/cancers Infections (bone tuberculosis, discitis) Congenital (e.g. spina bifida, dysplasia, deformations of the spine) Inflammation (e.g. osteoarthritis) Trauma (e.g. bone fractures)
Neurological disorders	Slipped disk with neurological symptoms Cervical myelopathy Cord compression Cauda equina syndrome
Vascular disorders	Heart attack Serious bleeding disorders (e.g. haemophilia, anticoagulation) Insufficiency/narrowing of the vertebral/carotid artery Vascular defects (e.g. aortic aneurysm)

Note: These cautions and contraindications are in addition to the general cautions and contraindications referred to for Tui Na in general.

Method

First, it is really important to understand that Ban Fa contains many hidden movements and postures that cannot be learned from a book or video alone, so learning Ban Fa must first be done in a class setting. Ban Fa is hugely about positioning of both the practitioner and the patient, and using tissue bindings and leverage to adjust the tissues. Ban Fa can be used on any joint, and there are many variations of Ban Fa depending on which part of the body you are applying it to, such as the neck, thoracic, lumbar, sacrum, shoulder, ankle, wrist or elbow. Below, I have written methods on how to adjust the cervical, thoracic and lumbar spine.

When performing Ban Fa, it is important to always use the patient's breath to apply the technique. Ask the patient to take a deep breath in, then perform Ban Fa as they breathe out. This puts the patient in a Yin state as the technique is performed, helping the tissues to be more relaxed and easier to manipulate without discomfort.

Ban Fa can and is largely used as an assisted stretch. *Do not perform overstretches or thrusts* until you have used Ban Fa as a stretch on many different people. This will enable you to become aware of a body's natural range of movement, and allow you to feel when it is right to apply Cun Jin (see above).

Both sides

Always perform Ban Fa on each side. If using Ban Fa as an assisted stretch, perform three times each side, and hold for 10–15 seconds. If applying Cun Jin, do this only once after two to three gentle assisted stretches.

颈椎扳法 Jing Zhui Ban Fa (cervical vertebra)

For safety reasons, the traditional method of Jing Zhui Ban Fa is not discussed in this book. This is due to the sensitive nature of the cervical vertebrae and the vertebral arteries that ascend through the transverse processes of the cervical spine. There are arguments both for and against the use of Ban Fa on the neck, and although if done correctly and for the correct indications it is very safe, the technique can still cause harm and is arguably unnecessary due to the amount of other techniques that can be performed in a much safer manner. That being said, the following is a method I have found to be much safer and, if the area is prepared well through other Tui Na techniques, has equally good results at mobilising the cervical vertebrae.

- With the patient sitting up, hold the occiput with your right hand, and place your left hand or left forearm on the patient's right jaw line.

- Tilt the head forward slightly to about 30 degrees (to take pressure away from the vertebral arteries), and rotate the head gently as far as it naturally goes to the left by pulling your left hand/arm and pushing your right hand.

- Hold it there for 10–15 seconds, and then let go quickly. Repeat on each side. If done correctly, the head should quickly spring back towards a neutral position causing a release of the neck tissues and mobilising the neck vertebrae.

- This can also be applied in the supine position with one hand on the occiput, and the other holding the patient's chin whilst applying a small amount of traction (Ba Shen Fa).

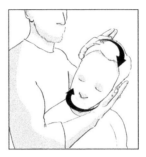

胸椎扳法 Xiong Zhui Ban Fa (thoracic vertebra)

There are many different versions of Xiong Zhui Ban Fa depending on what part of the thoracic you want to target, and also whether you want to manipulate with a thoracic twist, posterior pull or a thoracic lift.

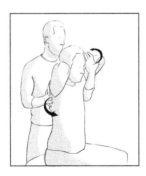 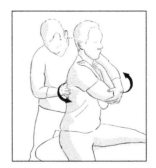

VERSION 1

- With the patient in a seated position on the bed or on a chair, stand behind them and ask the patient to place both hands with fingers interlaced behind their head.

- Place your knee or a rolled-up towel between the patient and yourself, and gently pull back their elbows.

- If using your knee, you can place your knee on the affected spine or just to the side, according to the affected area.

VERSION 2

- With the patient in a seated position, ask them to interlace their fingers, and put their hands in the air with their palms facing upwards whilst you stand behind them.

- Place your right hand on their back, at the level of the affected area, and then use your left hand/arm to bridge their arms.

- Push forwards with your right hand, and pull the patient's arms backwards to create an expansion of the chest. The heel of the right hand can be placed either on the spine or to the side of the spine.

VERSION 3

- With the patient in a seated position, stand behind them and ask the patient to place their hands on their opposite shoulders (so that their arms are crossed).

- If their left arm is over their right arm, reach around with your right hand and take a firm hold of their left elbow, slightly compressing their arm into their body.

- Place your left hand on their back, with the palm root to the left of their spine at the level that you wish to adjust. Your fingers should be facing outwards and your thumb facing up.

- Lean the patient forward ever so slightly, and begin to twist the patient's spine by pulling with your right hand whilst pushing with your left hand. This movement should be made from the legs and the hips, and your torso should move with the patient's torso for better stability.

- Rotate the patient as far as they feel is comfortable, then either hold for a few seconds and release quickly, or perform a quick overstretch/thrust within normal anatomical ranges.

- Repeat this on the other side with the patient's right arm over their left.

腰椎扳法 Yao Zhui Ban Fa (lumbar vertebra)

Yao Zhui Ban Fa is essentially the lumbar roll that is used in other systems such as Osteopathy or Chiropractic practice. Again, like many of the manipulations used within Tui Na, there are a couple of variations that we can use to adjust the patient's lumbar spine. However, the method detailed below is the stronger and more commonly used:

- Ask the patient to lay on their right side with both legs straight. Position the left leg bent, so that their left foot rests behind their right knee. It is important that their right leg is straight, to keep the spine in a neutral position.

- Gently pull the arm that is underneath the patient towards you to encourage the patient's torso to lie more horizontally, creating a slight twist in their spine. Occasionally this alone can manipulate the spine.

- Place your left hand/forearm on the patient's left shoulder and push towards the bed gently whilst pulling their left hip towards your hip with your right hand/forearm. Repeat on the other side.

- To focus on the upper lumbar or lower thoracic, place more emphasis on pushing the patient's shoulder whilst locking their hips in place. To focus on the patient's lower lumbar or lumbar-sacral joint, place more emphasis on the pulling of the patient's hip whilst locking their shoulders in place.

- Before attempting an overstretch/thrust, try rocking the patient with each hand/forearm slightly out of phase. This can sometimes have the same effect with much less force.

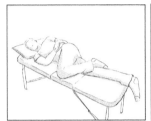 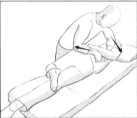

摇法 Yao Fa (rocking/rotating)

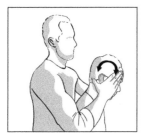

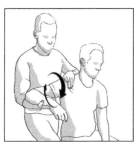

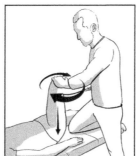

Technique category
Passive joint manipulation

Stages of treatment
Treatment stage

Therapeutic actions
Yao Fa lubricates joints, improves function and range of movement, removes obstruction and invigorates flow of Qi and Blood.

Yao Fa is the technique used to articulate a joint. Yao means to 'rotate, rock or row', and is essentially assisted movement, in which the practitioner passively puts a joint through assisted motion within its natural range of movement. Yao Fa can be performed on any joint, and must be done within the patient's natural and comfortable range of movement. This technique is commonly done on the joints of the limbs, neck and lumbar area.

Method

When performing Yao Fa, it is first of all important that you have secure hold of the patient's limb or body part. This is both so that the patient can fully relax and feel comfortable, and also so that you, as the practitioner, do not injure yourself with poor posture. This is especially the case with heavier body parts such as the legs.

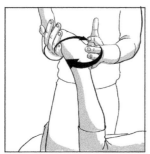

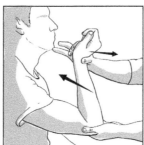

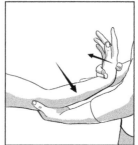

- When taking hold of the patient's body part that you wish to articulate, do so in a gentle manner so that the patient does not feel threatened and tense up. Take the whole weight of the body part in your hands.

- Begin moving the body part throughout its normal anatomical range, constantly 'listen' for any discomfort or restrictions from the patient.

- Movements can be in a two-dimensional or a three-dimensional plane, such as rocking or rotating respectively. Movements should start off small, and slowly increase in amplitude.

- Ensure that the patient is completely relaxed and not assisting with any movement.

Tips

- When performing Yao Fa, alternate between small and large ranges of movement.

- Perform Yao Fa smoothly and sensitively, never committing to strong movements.

- The patient must be completely relaxed to disengage any muscles.

TREATMENT GUIDELINES

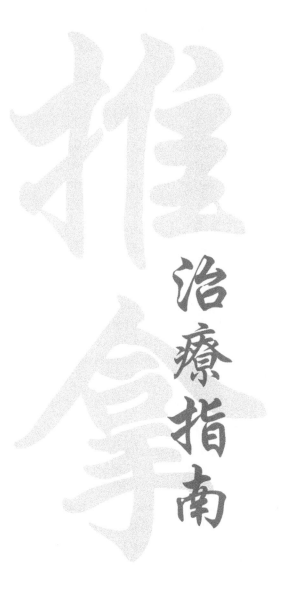

Chapter 10

Treatment Guidelines

The purpose of this section is not simply to give protocols or routines for specific conditions, but to hopefully give ideas, thoughts and considerations of how to treat each type of condition so that you will feel able to treat conditions that have not been specifically outlined in this book – as the Chinese proverb goes, 'It is better to teach a man to fish than to give him a fish' (*Shou Ren Yi Yu Bu Ru Shou Zhi Yi Yu*, 授人以魚不如授之以漁).

Don't get stuck!

Each treatment and Tui Na routine should be *spontaneous*. Do not use a *prescription* or *routine* simply because 'it worked last time'. If it *worked* last time, it means that the patient's condition has *changed*, and therefore so should the treatment!

I am a huge believer that each treatment and Tui Na routine should be spontaneous. The routines in this chapter are basic, giving you a rough idea of how to treat specific conditions, and should act simply as a guide at the beginning of your study and practice. Treatment should always be based entirely on the individual and their diagnosis should not have any preconceived ideas or prescriptions before the consultation itself. That is not to say don't be prepared, but don't have ideas set in stone such as 'the patient has booked in with anxiety, so when I see them I will do this and that'. It is also important to not use a prescription simply because 'it worked last time'. If it worked last time, it means that the patient's condition has changed, and therefore so should the treatment!

Stages of treatment

Whilst carrying out any treatment, no matter how long or how short, it is important to take it through the three key stages of treatment – essentially like any good story it will have a beginning, a middle and an end. Each stage needs to be in place for the treatment to be both effective and to help the body to adapt to the changes that are taking place during and after the treatment. For instance, if we were to begin a treatment with heavy techniques that work on the deeper layers of the body, the patient's tissues will likely fight back. This will create tension, pain and damage, and perhaps even make the patient's condition worse. However, if we were to spend time opening and warming the channels, allowing the patient's body to adapt to the changes that are occurring over the course of the session, the patient's body is more likely to yield and be receptive to any transformations that need to take place. The following are the three key stages of treatment.

Opening stage

The first stage of treatment is known as the 'opening stage'. During this first stage, you are introducing yourself to the body whilst also relaxing both yourself and the patient. It is called the 'opening stage' because you are opening the channels in order to allow an optimal flow of Qi, Blood and Body Fluids throughout the body, particularly to the area that you are focusing on. This stage is performed on the Wei Qi (superficial) level, starting off superficially and gradually penetrating deeper. It is essential to start at this stage as to not cause the patient to fight back by tensing, or even going into spasm.

Considerations

- Connect to the patient.

- Sink your intention through your hands and into the patient.

- Relax both the patient and yourself.

- Open the Sinew channels.

Tips

- The more relaxed you are, the more relaxed the patient will be.

- Where the mind (Yi) goes, the Qi follows. Keep your eyes open and your focus on what you are doing and trying to achieve.

Treatment stage

Now that you have moved progressively deeper into the body with both technique and intention, this is the stage at which you are treating the patient and having a therapeutic effect. Now that you have worked on the Wei level, this stage has an effect on the Ying and Yuan levels of Qi. This stage also allows you to manipulate and align the Sinew channels with more permanent affect. During the treatment stage, you can also palpate for further diagnosis at a deeper level if you wish, as any tension caused by the body 'guarding' itself should now have been reduced. Techniques should be performed deeper (according to constitution and disease) for therapeutic results, and the use of acupressure will be more affective due to the Sinew channels being activated and opened during the first stage. It is a good idea to use three to five acupressure points (a combination of local and distal) during this stage to stimulate the body's energetic system and natural self-healing mechanisms. Stronger techniques such as **An Fa/Ya Fa** and **Tan Bo Fa** may be used once this stage is fully established, in addition to point-stimulating techniques such as **Yi Zhi Chan Tui Fa**. It is at the *end* of this stage that manipulative techniques such as **Ba Shen Fa** and **Ban Fa** should be used.

Considerations

- Use stronger techniques to penetrate deeper.

- Choose to use three to five acupressure points that aim to treat the main complaint.

- Perform manipulations and passive movement if required.

Tips

- Techniques such as **Gun Fa** and **Rou Fa** are excellent at bridging the gap between the opening stage and treatment stage due to their adaptive nature.

Closing stage

The third and final stage of treatment is called the 'closing stage', and is also known as the 'dispersing stage'. Once the treatment stage has been completed, it is important to use techniques to remove any stagnations that may have been created during the treatment, and to also bring the patient back into a more conscious and invigorated state. Dispersing techniques such as **Dou Fa**, **Ji Fa** and **Pai Fa** are commonly used at this stage. **Tui Fa** is also used at the end to dredge the patient's Jing Luo system and to direct the flow of Qi downwards to have a grounding effect. These specific techniques are also very therapeutic for the practitioner at the end of treatment due to the shaking and stretching nature of performing the techniques.

Considerations

- It is important to use dispersing techniques during this stage to both bring the patient back from a semi-conscious state, and also to resolve any stagnation that may have been caused during the treatment.

Tip

- Use this stage to also dredge yourself at the end of treatment.

Left or right, up or down?

When learning Tui Na, a common question is often, 'which side do I start on, and which direction should I go?' Generally speaking, when treating the limbs, treatment should focus on the torso and then towards the affected limb first and foremost (sometimes only one limb is necessary unless the other limbs are compensating), whereas when treating conditions of the main trunk of the body, treatment should focus on both sides so that balance is achieved.

In regards to deciding which side to start on, unless the patient's discomfort or pain dictates otherwise, it was classically said that treatment should begin on the left side for males and on the right side for females. This is due to the directional movement of Qi within the female and male energetic system. If the patient is experiencing severe pain, however, and they are too sensitive to receive treatment on the side of the injury, it is a good idea to begin treatment on the opposite side so that the treatment draws the attention away from the injured site.

When deciding to work either up or down the body, this depends on the state of the Qi and Blood within the body. Generally speaking, we work in the direction that we desire the Qi and Blood to flow. For instance, if a patient presents with a condition where the Qi is descending and sinking more than it should, we would start treatment at the lower parts of the body and work upwards. We would treat vice versa when a patient presented with a condition caused by the Qi ascending and rising. Whichever way the treatment is performed, however, it is important for the treatment to finish with a downward directional movement. This is because Qi naturally rises, yet the safest way for Qi to flow is downward. We essentially need to keep grounded, like an electrical circuit.

Grounding the patient

Qi naturally rises, yet the safest way for Qi to travel is down. No matter what direction the Qi has been guided during treatment, it is always a good idea to spend at least a few seconds at the end of each treatment to 'ground the Qi'.

Treatment of common conditions

It is important to understand that Tui Na is designed to be a whole medical system, and that musculoskeletal conditions are only part of its ability (although a major part due to the physical and external nature of Tui Na). The following chapters cover the major fields of both internal and external medicine:

- Mental/emotional disorders.

- Respiratory disorders.

- Digestive disorders.

- Gynaecology disorders.

- Muskuloskeletal disorders.

The chapters focus on the key principles and considerations to take within each field, followed by general treatment suggestions. When treating Tui Na as a whole medical system, it is obviously vital that it is also treated with the respect of a whole medical system, and that with each and every treatment a full Chinese Medicine consultation and diagnosis is taken. With this in mind, the following pages (alongside a full Chinese Medicine diagnosis) should provide a solid platform for which to build a treatment plan for your patients.

Chapter 11

Mental/Emotional Disorders

Within Chinese Medicine, it is considered that the main energetic function of each of the Primary channels is to assist in the processing of specific psychological aspects of the mind. For example, it is known that Grief and Melancholy pertain to the Lungs. It is the function of the Lung channel to facilitate the processing of Grief, and to enable the body to smoothly progress through the process of grieving. If there is stagnation within the Lung channel, the grieving process will not be smooth – there may be lack of acknowledgment of Grief with a risk of storing the emotion of Grief and not moving forward properly. The Large Intestine channel, on the other hand, has the function of enabling the body to 'let go' of stored emotions, in addition to other attachments such as those to a situation, material belongings or cravings and addictions. Again, regulating and ensuring a free flow of Qi and Blood through the Large Intestine channel will facilitate this action, and enable the letting go of emotions and attachments. A list of all channels and their functions in regards to the psyche can be seen below.

Channel	Psychological function	Psychological dysfunction
Lung	To experience and release emotions, especially grief, loss and melancholy	Inability to release emotions, and feeling numb to grief or loss
Large Intestine	To assist in the letting go of emotion and attachments	Inability to let go of a situation, emotion or an attachment
Stomach	To process and 'digest' our thoughts and ideas	Inability to put thoughts into action
Spleen	To receive information and generate thoughts and ideas	Inability to think clearly and generate ideas
Heart	To process the emotions of joy and heartache, and to develop intimate relationships	Inability to process sadness and heartbreak, and inability to express
Small Intestine	To provide the ability of discernment, and to know what is both good and bad for ourselves and others	Inability to make decisions that are good for ourselves, and inability to separate the important from the unimportant
Bladder	To give self-worth and to process our insecurities	Low self-esteem and self-worth

Channel	Psychological function	Psychological dysfunction
Kidney	To process both rational and irrational fears, and to establish our connection with Ming	Paranoia, phobias and the general feeling of intimidation; also the feeling that 'nothing seems to go right for me'
Pericardium	To act as protection to the Heart from excessive emotions	Inability to keep people emotionally at a distance, or inability to let people in
San Jiao	To assist with integration and the development of social relations	Inability to develop social relationships and to integrate with others
Gall Bladder	To assist in decision-making and to give the courage to externalise and realise those decisions	Inability to make a decision or externalise a decision
Liver	To process the emotions of anger and frustration, and to assist with drive and ambition	Feeling of frustration and becoming easily irritated; lack of drive and vision for ambition

Although it is the function of the Primary channels to deal with the above psychological aspects of the mind, treating and regulating the associated Sinew channels can and will have a beneficial effect on the flow of Qi and Blood within the Primary channels. This will help with the regulation of the emotions and psychological aspects of the mind. The relationships between the channels and the psyche should be considered when treating all conditions, but especially when treating disorders of the mind. Equally, it is important for the body to have 'space' for Qi and Blood to flow, and it is largely the Sinew channels that control the space within the body in regards to causing contraction and relaxation. For instance, by treating the Lung and Pericardium Sinew channels, we can open up the chest cavity to allow better circulation of Qi and Blood around the Lungs and the Heart. This helps with the processing and expression of emotion due to the functions of the Lung and Heart organs and channels. Equally, treating the Bladder Sinew channel and encouraging better upright posture can offer the patient better self-esteem and self-confidence by helping them to 'stand tall'.

When consulting patients with mental/emotional conditions, it can be difficult to get the true story from the patient in regards to how they are feeling. In some countries (I'm talking from experience within the UK), it is very unnatural for people to share their feelings, and can be difficult when meeting someone for the first time. When asking how the patient is emotionally, or how they are coping with things, it is often very useful to watch their body language rather than listen to their words. For instance:

- Do they answer your question abruptly (relating to Liver)?

- Does their head tilt downwards slightly when they talk about themselves (Bladder)?

- Do they sink a little with a sunken chest when they say that they feel 'fine' (relating to Lung)?

There are many observational signs that are useful when asking about how the patient is feeling, and it is important to take note of their movements.

The Five Spirits (Wu Shen, 五神)

When discussing mental/emotional disorders, it would be wrong to not mention the Wu Shen (五神). If we want to successfully diagnose or treat mental/emotional disorders from a Chinese Medicine perspective, we need to understand the Wu Shen in depth. However, this is a brief summary here, as a small section of a chapter could never do justice to the complex and in-depth nature of Shen.

The concept of Shen, which can be further split into the Wu Shen, is fundamentally the study of the psyche and the aspects of the mind within Chinese Medicine. The Shen is one of the Three Treasures, and is the collective term for the human spirit – essentially, a patient 'without Shen' will not recover. Shen is the most refined of the Vital Substances (it is Qi on the verge of becoming consciousness), and is what forms the basis and foundation of human consciousness. Shen can be split into five aspects, known as the Wu (five) Shen (Spirit), with each of them relating to a different facet of the psyche. Each of the five Shen rarely work in isolation, and all human thought and consciousness is based on a combination of the Wu Shen.

Note: Shen can be used for both the collective term for the Five Spirits (Wu Shen) in addition to the one Shen (related to the Heart) that is discussed first below.

Shen (神, mind/consciousness)

The Shen is the most Yang of the Five Spirits, and is the spirit that connects us to and communicates with the Heavens/Yuan Shen/Dao. It is often interpreted as our mind, and is considered to govern our consciousness. The Shen is thought to reside within the centre of the Heart, and is said to flow from the orifices of the Heart within the Blood. In Chinese Medicine, when referring to the centre of the Heart, it does not literally mean the spaces within the physical structure of the Heart, but actually within the spaces and stillness within consciousness. This is important to understand, as generally it is only when there is stillness within the consciousness (when the patient is relaxed, at ease and comfortable) that the Shen can be treated effectively.

It is from within the Heart, and the Blood, that the Shen helps to guide us along our path and gives us our self-identity. When the Shen is healthy, there will be good self-awareness, insight and inspiration. The emotions will flow freely from the 'orifices of the Heart', and there will be good emotional expression.

The main manifestation of the Shen is through the eyes. Although Shen is invisible, a healthy Shen can be seen by a brightness that shines from the eyes, and the ability to connect with someone through the eyes. Generally, treatment of the Shen should involve promoting circulation (especially between the head and the body), nourishing the vessels and treating the Pericardium. The key functions and dysfunctions of the Shen can be found below:

Key functions of the Shen (神)

- Provides the ability to think clearly and sharply.

- Provides the ability to sleep soundly.

- Provides self-awareness.

- Provides intelligence in conjunction with the Yi and the Zhi.

- Provides insight and intuition through connection to the Yuan Shen.

- Provides emotional expression.

- Assists in memory (particularly skills) alongside the Yi and the Zhi.

- Provides wisdom (in conjunction with the Zhi).

Key symptoms of Shen (神) disorders

- Being overly talkative or speaking incoherently.

- Lack of self-awareness.

- Insomnia.

- Dream-disturbed sleep.

- Drifting in and out of consciousness (in extreme cases).

- Lack of concentration.

- Mania and mental restlessness.

Hun (魂, ethereal soul)

The Hun is the Yang aspect of the soul, and is said to leave the body after death and return to the heavens. There are, in fact, three Hun within Daoism, although they are generally discussed as one within Chinese Medicine.

It is said that 'the Liver houses the Hun' – the Hun likes to wander freely, and is anchored within the Liver Blood. The Hun represents our vision, imagination and ability to see our true path. It is the spirit that gives us our ambition and goals, and enables us to plan and strategise. The Hun essentially gives the Shen direction through its vision.

When the Hun is constrained, it is thought to get 'angry', as the Hun prefers to wander freely and does not like to become stuck (through Qi and Blood stagnation, for instance). If the Hun is what we call 'wrong', then it can become rebellious, whereas when it is corrected, it will obey. Rebellion is simply a way that the body is trying to correct itself from the feeling of suppression. Once the source of suppression is addressed, the Hun will become less rebellious. Treatment of the Hun should be through the Blood, more specifically, the Liver Blood, in order to anchor and nourish the Hun. Also having freedom and space to go about things is important to regulate the Hun. Movement helps, with stretching and opening the joints being particularly good to soothe the Hun by allowing the Qi and Blood to flow freely.

Key functions of the Hun (魂)

- Provides vision, both physically (through the eyes) and mentally (via dreams and ambitions).

- Provides direction to the Shen.

- Provides rational thinking and decision-making.

- Provides the ability to make plans and carry them forward.

- Provides the courage to take action and externalise thoughts.

Key symptoms of Hun (魂) disorders

- Depression.

- Insomnia, with dream-disturbed sleep or nightmares.

- Repressed emotions.

- Recklessness.

- Timidity.

- Aimlessness and lack of direction.

- Lack of vision (both physically and psychologically).

- Closed-mindedness and stubbornness.

- Rebellion and frustration.

- Angry or irritable outbursts.

Po (魄, corporeal soul)

The Po represent the Yin soul, which is the soul that returns to the Earth upon death. The Po are a group of seven spirits that are said to reside in the Lungs (due to the breath helping to regulate the Po), and make up the primitive aspect to our soul. They are therefore thought to be related to the primitive aspects of our brain such as the limbic system, and also our autonomic nervous system. The Po are responsible for our physical sensations, such as touch, in addition to our emotional sensations, such as 'feeling' sad. Essentially, it is through the Po that we can experience life. The Po are sometimes referred to as our 'animal soul', and give us our animal wit and sense of 'knowing'.

Due to the fact that the Po are first to experience the world around us, they also create our physical and emotional attachments to it. This can lead to cravings and addictions, both physically and mentally, and the storing of emotions that have arisen from past experiences and events. (Storing of emotions is also discussed briefly in Chapter 13 on digestive disorders, due to the fact that the digestive system generally acts as the repository of our unresolved emotions.) If our Po are disturbed, we will have addictive personalities or develop unhealthy attachments. It is the Po that also enable us to let go and move on, both from these attachments and our emotions. The attachments that Po may be affected by are as follows:

- Pleasures and indulgences
- Anger and resentment
- Worries and fears
- Sadness and loss
- Likes and dislikes
- Objects and ownerships
- Sexual desires.

Treatment of the Po should be through nourishment of the Zong Qi, which is the Qi that is formed within the chest, and to connect the Lungs to the Kidneys in order to 'ground' or 'anchor' them. Due to the Po's relationship with the Lungs, regulating the breath is a good way to treat disorders of the Po, and deep breathing is important to 'draw the Lungs down to the Kidneys'.

Key functions of the Po (魄)

- Provides mindfulness and the ability to be in the now.
- Provides the ability to feel (physically and emotionally).
- Provides the ability to let go of attachments.
- Regulates autonomic functions such as heart rate, breathing and peristalsis.

Key symptoms of Po (魄) disorders

- Asthma and breathing difficulties.
- Bowel disorders (most commonly constipation).
- Chronic tension or pain.
- Cravings and addictions.
- Eating disorders.
- Extreme reactions or lack of reactions to sadness.
- Feelings of unease and discomfort.
- Obsessions (including obsessive-compulsive disorder, OCD).

Zhi (志, willpower/drive)

The Zhi is said to be our motivation, drive and our willpower. It is the most Yin of the spirits and therefore the most dense, and resides deep within the Kidneys and Jing. Due to it being the most Yin of the Shen, naturally one of its functions is also to root the other four Shen. The term Zhi (志) is also used for the word 'memory', and is the spirit that acts in conjunction with the Shen and the Yi to help with the storage of memories (in particular, the memories of events).

If the Zhi is disturbed, we may lose our drive or motivation do get things done. On the other hand, there may be 'too much' willpower, which is an excess condition that may cause people to try to 'force' an outcome even when every sign is telling them it should not happen. Due to the Zhi being housed in the Kidneys, treatment of the Zhi is based around nourishing and consolidating Jing, and the Kidney Qi should be anchored and protected.

Key functions of the Zhi (志)

- Provides willpower, motivation and drive.
- Assists in memory (particularly events) in conjunction with the Shen and Yi.
- Provides wisdom (in conjunction with the Shen).
- Provides congenital intelligence.
- Assists in the connection to Ming (destiny) and our life path.

Key symptoms of Zhi (志) disorders

- Forgetfulness.
- Lack of motivation or 'get up and go'.
- Inability to kick habits.
- Depression.
- Rational and irrational fears.
- Low self-esteem and self-worth.
- The feeling of 'nothing ever goes right for me'.

Yi (意, intellect/thought)

The Yi is the aspect of our spirit that is related to our intellect, focus and intention. It is said to be housed by the Spleen, and is therefore directly affected by the quality of our diet. The Yi gives us our thoughts, actions and mental clarity – it is our acquired intelligence. Like the Earth in the centre of the other elements, the Yi is at the centre of the Five Spirits, and acts as the 'spiritual pivot' between them that helps to put the other spirits into action, allows them to communicate and allows us to apply them.

It is said that if the Yi is strong, the mind will be clear and ideas will generate. The mind will be focused and will have the ability to concentrate on tasks for longer periods. However, if the Yi is weak (for instance, due to poor diet), then thinking will be slow and dull, and the ability to learn and memorise will also be poor. Due to the Yi's relationship with the Spleen, treatment of the Yi should be focused around treating the Ying Qi and the overall constitution of the patient. Diet is an extremely important factor when regulating the Yi.

Key functions of the Yi (意)

- Generates thoughts and new ideas.

- Enables the application of our thoughts and psychological processes.

- Provides focus and intent.

- Assists in concentration and study.

- Assists in the development of our acquired intelligence.

- Assists in memory (particularly facts) in conjunction with the Shen and Zhi.

Key symptoms of Yi (意) disorders

- Obsessive thoughts and worries.

- Clouded thinking and mind 'fog'.

- Lack of concentration.

- Inability to think clearly.

- Inability to take action on thoughts or ideas.

- Knotted feeling within the abdomen.

- Impaired digestion, made worse with worry.

Ultimately, when seeing patients with mental/emotional disorders, it is first and foremost important to identify both the emotion(s) involved in addition to understanding the current balance of their psyche as well as the patient's pattern according to syndrome differentiation. Once it has been distinguished which of the Wu Shen are out of balance and which of the Seven Emotions are excessive, we are then able to choose which channels need to be checked and treated in order to restore balance to the emotions and the mind. Treating the corresponding channels can help to process and release any stored emotions, and also help to balance the Wu Shen to regulate the mind.

Treatment to regulate the Shen (神)

When looking to treat the Shen, it is important that the patient is completely relaxed and comfortable so that their Shen can regulate within the stillness of their consciousness. If there is disruption within the treatment room or outside, or if the patient does not feel content and relaxed in any way, the Shen will not be reached and the treatment will have an affect only on the Qi and Blood rather than the Shen itself.

Engaging the Heart

During treatment, it is important for patient to have a gentle smile that pulls slightly on the corners of their mouth, as this pulls on the fascia surrounding the Heart. By smiling, the Heart will become engaged and the spaces within the chest will begin to open. This allows better circulation of Heart Qi within the chest, and through the Heart channels. You can experience this for yourself – by simply smiling for around 30 seconds, you will begin to feel happy and experience a warm feeling in and around the chest area.

It is also useful to explain this to your patient as an after-care advice 'exercise', and suggest that they smile throughout the day for 20–30 seconds at a time, even if they do not feel happy, as this can create movement of the Heart Qi and thus create a feeling of joy. This is a simple way of expression, which strengthens the Fire element and therefore the Shen.

Perform the following base treatment to prepare the body for regulating the Shen and calming the mind:

- Begin with performing gentle **Ba Shen Fa** on each of the limbs in addition to gentle **Ba Shen Fa** on the head and neck to allow Qi and Blood to flow through the Qi Men.

- Open the 'Gates of Consciousness' (see page 223) by using **An Fa** and **Rou Fa** on DU-16 (Feng Fu), BL-10 (Tian Zhu), and GB-20 (Feng Chi) each, for around one to two minutes.

- Release the tongue by placing your thumb and first two fingers either side of the tongue root (externally) underneath the patient's chin. This stimulates the point EX-M-HN-20 (Yu Ye/Jin Jin) externally. Perform a **Nian Fa** type action with a comfortable upward force (towards the root of the tongue) to release the tongue. This is sometimes called 'Twin Dragons Play with Pearls'.

- Use **An Fa** on the palm of the hands, focusing on P-8 (Lao Gong), followed by **Fen Tui Fa** on the palms and at the palm root. This is known as separating Yin and Yang and helps to open Lao Gong. Use **Yi Zhi Chan Tui Fa** on R-17 (Shan Zhong) to help activate the Pericardium and to open the Chest to help release emotion.

The mirror to the Heart

The tongue is the mirror to the Heart, and releasing the tongue externally by using **Nian Fa** at the tongue root beneath the chin can help to open and vent excess Qi from the Heart. This technique is known as 'Twin Dragons Play with Pearls', and can have a profound effect on patients with excess Qi in the chest, causing conditions such as anxiety, insomnia and/or palpitations.

The Seven Emotions (七情, Qi Qing)

According to Chinese Medicine, all internal causes of disease are due to one or more of what are known as the Seven Emotions (Qi Qing, 七情). These are the basic emotions that arise as by-products from interactions of the mind and both our internal and external environment. Each one has a very specific effect on an organ, a channel (as mentioned above) and the flow of Qi. They are essentially internal pathogens, and although it is considered perfectly normal (and healthy) to have an emotion, it is absolutely necessary to vent and to purge any emotion that arises (before it causes damage within the body).

When the mind reacts to an internal or external stimulus, certain emotions will emerge depending on the balance of the mind. When we experience an emotion, what we are really feeling is fluctuations in the movement and quality of Qi. Each emotion has its own movement and quality: Anger has a different quality to Grief, which is different to Sadness, Worry or Fear and so on. When we experience an emotion strongly enough, or for long enough, that deviation in quality and movement of Qi can affect the whole body and alter the physical tissues of the body, especially the Sinew channels. If we allow the emotions to last for hours or days, we may simply call it a feeling or a mood. This occurs at the Wei level, and will affect the Sinew channels in terms of contraction or relaxation. When the emotion is unresolved and lasts for weeks or months, it moves to the Ying level and becomes a temperament. This begins to affect the way our Qi and Blood flows throughout our bodies. When this emotion becomes trapped and lasts even longer, such as years, it moves to the Yuan level and becomes stored within our deeper vessels such as the Divergent channels and/or our Extraordinary Vessels (particularly the Chong Mai). These emotions can be perceived as a personality trait. The Seven Emotions, their corresponding organ/channel and their effects on the flow of Qi can be found in the table below:

Seven Emotions	Organ/ channel*	Effect on the Qi flow
Anger (怒, Nu)	Liver	Causes the Qi to quickly ascend
Grief (悲, Bei)	Lung	Causes the Qi to be drastically consumed
Anxiety (憂, You)	Lung and Heart	Causes the Qi to become blocked in the upper Jiao
Joy/Excitement (喜, Xi)	Heart	Causes the Qi to slow down and slacken
Worry/Pensiveness (思, Si)	Spleen	Causes the Qi to knot in the middle Jiao
Fear/Dread (恐, Kong)	Kidney	Causes the Qi to descend
Shock (驚, Jing)	Heart and Kidney	Causes the Qi to scatter and the Jing to freeze

* It is important to be flexible with the organs that the emotions can affect. Any emotion can have some effect on any organ due to its effect on the Qi and Blood, and all emotions affect the Heart due to its function of housing the Shen, and to some extent the Liver, due to it being responsible for the free flowing of Qi (and therefore the emotions).

Treatment to regulate the emotions

When treating the emotions, before anything else, it is first necessary to address the overall quality and movement of Qi and Blood within the body. This can be an incredibly simple yet effective way to help neutralise specific emotions and allow the body to self-regulate. For instance, if there is Anger, which causes the Qi to quickly rise, we can simply encourage the Qi to descend. Conversely, if there is Fear, which causes the Qi to descend, we can use Tui Na to help ascend the Qi. If the Qi is knotted, we can use techniques to help unknot the Qi, whereas if the Qi has been scattered by Fright or Shock, we can use techniques to gather the Qi. This should be done before anything else, as more often than not, correcting the quality and movement of Qi within the body can rectify the emotional state of the patient. Below are examples of ways to treat each emotion by correcting the movement and quality of Qi.

Anger (怒, Nu)

Anger causes the Qi to quickly rise, and is attributed to the Wood element and the Liver. The goal is therefore to descend the Qi and regulate the Liver Sinew channels. We can do this by asking the patient to lie on their front in prone position. Start by using **Mo Fa** on the back, followed by **Tui Fa** down the Bladder Sinew channel 36 times. Use **Fen Tui Fa** across the Bladder Sinew channels on the upper back and shoulders to relax the tissues. Ask the patient to take a deep breath in, and use **An Fa** to stimulate GB-21 (Jian Jing) as they breathe out. The patient should then hold their breath *out* for 3–4 seconds whilst GB-21 (Jian Jing) is being stimulated. Repeat this for six breaths. Ask the patient to turn over and lie on their back in a supine position. Use **Tui Fa** to push down the Ren Mai from R-22 (Tian Tu) to R-12 (Zhong Wan). Repeat this 36 times. This helps to root the Qi within the Ren Mai, which will descend the Qi and Blood. Use combinations of **Gun Fa**, **Rou Fa** and **An Fa** along the Liver Sinew channel in a downward movement to help open and regulate the Liver channel, and finish off by using **An Fa** on K-1 (Yong Quan) and Lv-3 (Tai Chong) to draw down the Qi. Again, ask the patient to breathe deeply and hold their breath *out* for 3–4 seconds each time. This should be repeated six times for each point. Holding the breath out helps to bring the body into a state of Yin, creating space and stillness.

Grief (悲, Bei)

Grief causes the Qi to be consumed or depleted, especially of the Lungs, so we therefore need to gather and tonify the Qi and regulate the Lung channels. We can do this by asking the patient to lie in a supine position. Use **Yi Zhi Chan Tui Fa** to stimulate LU-1 (Zhong Fu) on both sides of the body to draw Qi inwards and towards the chest. Whilst stimulating LU-1 (Zhong Fu), ask the patient to take a deep breath, and hold their breath *in* for 4–5 seconds. Holding the breath in helps to bring the body into a state of Yang, giving a tonifying action within the chest (where the breath is held). Repeat this nine times. Next, use **Mo Fa** on the upper abdomen, and again use **Yi Zhi Chan Tui Fa** to stimulate R-12 (Zhong Wan) to gather Qi within the abdomen and chest, and R-6 (Qi Hai) to activate the Dan Tian to tonify and mobilise the Qi. In a seated position, perform **Cuo Fa** down the arms, focusing on the Lung Sinew channel. Repeat this nine times, followed by using **Rou Fa** with the thumb to stimulate LU-3 (Tian Fu) and LU-9 (Tai Yuan) for 1–2 minutes each.

Anxiety (憂, You)

Anxiety causes the Qi to become blocked in the upper Jiao, and is often attributed to the Lungs and the Heart. We therefore need to open the chest and unblock the Qi to allow it to flow in and out of the upper Jiao. Do this by placing your hands on the patient's ribcage, with your thumbs sitting just underneath, facing each other, as if to begin performing **Fen Tui Fa**. As the patient breathes in, press the thumbs underneath the ribs and into the diaphragm. As the patient breathes out, shake and vibrate the thumbs to help release the diaphragm. This should be repeated for 3–5 breaths. Once the diaphragm has been released, use **An Fa** to press down on GB-21 (Jian Jing) as the patient breathes out. Repeat this six times. With the patient in a seated position, use **An Fa** or **Rou Fa** with the thumb to stimulate P-6 (Nei Guan) for 1–2 minutes to open up the chest, followed by **Tui Fa** from P-7 (Da Ling) to P-3 (Qu Ze) to open up the Pericardium channel. Use **Na Fa** on the nape of the neck to relieve tension around the occiput whilst stimulating GB-20 (Feng Chi). Finish by using **Cuo Fa** on the intercostals for 1–2 minutes.

Joy/Excitement (喜, Xi)

Joy/excitement causes the Qi and Blood to slacken and to slow down due to the Fire element (of which Joy is attributed to), causing expansion within the vessels. Therefore, we need to 'tighten' the Qi and speed up the movement of Qi. 'Tightening' the Qi should be done by causing the tissues and vessels to contract slightly. This can be achieved by adding a little more pressure than would usually be necessary (as discussed in Section 3). By adding more pressure to the techniques, the body tissues contract as a method of defence, and the blood pressure will rise slightly, causing the Qi and Blood to flow more quickly.

Worry/Pensiveness (思, Si)

Worry/pensiveness causes the Qi to knot, and primarily affects the middle Jiao due to the location of the Stomach and Spleen. Therefore, we need to unknot the Qi and regulate the middle Jiao. We can do this by performing **Mo Fa** followed by **Rou Fa** on the abdomen. This helps to create space within the abdomen through relaxation and allows the Yi to become unobstructed. Use **Yi Zhi Chan Tui Fa** to stimulate R-12 (Zhong Wan) and SP-21 (Da Bao) to help unravel and unbind the Qi respectively. Use a combination of **An Fa** (with the palm), **Rou Fa** and **Gun Fa** down the leg aspects of the Spleen and Stomach Sinew channels to help open and regulate the channels and to assist in processing thoughts and worries by regulating the Yi. Finish off by using **An Fa** or **Rou Fa** with the thumb to stimulate ST-36 (Zu San Li), Lv-3 (Tai Chong) and SP-3 (Tai Bai) for 1–2 minutes each. Since diet is also an important factor in treating Worry/Pensiveness, it is essential to make adequate changes to the diet if needed.

Fear/Dread (恐, Kong)

Fear/dread causes the Qi to descend, so we therefore need to help the Qi to rise. We can do this by first using **Ca Fa** and/or **Tui Fa** in an upwards direction along the Du channel to activate and rise Yang Qi. Use **Na Fa** at the nape of the neck to relax and open the region of the occiput, followed by stimulating DU-16 (Feng Fu) with **An Fa** or **Rou Fa**. Use **Gun Fa** and **Rou Fa** on the lower back, focusing on BL-23 (Shen Shu) and BL-52 (Zhi Shi). Stimulate K-6 (Zhao Hai) with **Rou Fa** to raise Qi (through the Yin Qiao Mai), SP-6 (San Yin Jiao) to assist the Spleen in ascending the Qi, and finish off by stimulating DU-20 (Bai Hui) with **An Fa** or **Rou Fa** to again raise Yang.

Shock (驚, Jing)

Shock causes the Qi to scatter, so we therefore need to gather and root the Qi. We can do this by focusing on the Ren Mai and Kidney Sinew channel to help root the Qi, and use techniques and specific points to gather the Qi at each of the three Dan Tian. When treating Shock, it is best to start at the upper part of the body and work down, as this also helps to root the Qi. Begin with asking the patient to lie on their back in a relaxed supine position, and use **Ma Fa** to wipe from EX-M-HN-3 (Yin Tang) to DU-24 (Shen Ting) nine times, followed by gathering Qi at the upper Dan Tian by stimulating EX-M-HN-3 (Yin Tang) with **Rou Fa** for 1–2 minutes. Use **Ca Fa** from R-17 (Shan Zhong) to the navel 36 times, followed by gathering Qi at the middle Dan Tian by using **Yi Zhi Chan Tui Fa** to stimulate R-17 (Shan Zhong) for 1–2 minutes. Finally, use **Mo Fa** and **Rou Fa** on the lower abdomen for 1–2 minutes, followed by gathering Qi at the lower Dan Tian by gently using **Rou Fa** (with the thumb) to stimulate R-4 (Guan Yuan) for 1–2 minutes. Once Qi has been gathered at the three Dan Tian, use a combination of **An Fa**, **Gun Fa** and **Rou Fa** to work down the leg aspect of the Kidney Sinew channel to open and regulate the channel to help with the rooting of Qi. Finish off by pressing and holding K-1 (Yuan Quan) for 1–2 minutes to draw the Qi down.

As mentioned in the introduction to mental/emotional disorders (see page 209), should the body be open and the channels functioning properly, our emotions will be processed efficiently and our mind can carry on as normal – in a neutral setting, if you like. However, if the body is unable to process the emotion, it will become stuck and the emotion will be stored within the body. The type or strength of the emotion will dictate the way in which the body stores the emotion and where. To begin with, storing an emotion may not cause too much of an issue and may go unnoticed. However, the longer it is stored for, and as the amount of emotion that is being stored becomes greater, it will become more and more of an issue. For instance, if someone has an experience that makes them feel sad and they are unable to process that sadness (perhaps due to having to stay strong for others), they will store it within their body and most likely their Sinew channels. Over time, that person will react to situations with sadness or even with a sense of hopelessness due to the nature of sadness affecting their Po. As time goes on, the sadness will become greater and deeper if not dealt with. The emotions become buried within the Divergent and Extraordinary channels. The person will now not only react to situations from a place of sadness, but begin to perceive the world through an illusion or bias of sadness based on their stored emotion before any situation even takes place. This is how people manage to cause events based on their current and even past emotional state. Of course, this can happen with any of the seven core emotions, and will affect people in various different ways.

'Letting go'

It can often be difficult for the patient to be able to 'let go' and change certain mindsets. This may not necessarily be a conscious realisation. Our mind is made up of two major parts: the 'acquired mind' and the 'congenital mind'. It is the role of the acquired mind to experience, learn and to store. The acquired mind feels that for every experience it goes through, it must learn from it and store the lesson for the next time a similar situation arises. This is essentially wisdom, and is vital to the process of survival. However, more often than not, there is an emotion attached to each 'lesson'. What we end up with is the acquired mind 'storing' certain emotions and feelings from previous situations and events that may not be useful, but may also be detrimental. However, when it comes to 'letting go' of these emotions, we are basically telling the acquired mind that it was 'wrong' to have stored those emotions in the first place. As the acquired mind does not like being 'wrong' (some more than others, depending on the balance within mind and also the 'ego'), it can make it difficult to let go of an emotion and/or change a mindset. Some patients will seem stubborn and find it difficult to alter the paradigm of the mind, no matter how accurate the treatment. Based on the concept of the psyche within Chinese Medicine, this largely comes down to the Po and its attachments. This is covered above, in the discussion on the Wu Shen (Five Spirits).

Key acupressure points

BL-42 (Po Hu), BL-44 (Shen Tang), BL-47 (Hun Men), BL-49 (Yi She) and **BL-52 (Zhi Shi)** on the outer Bladder channel all have an effect on the Wu Shen, affecting the Po, Shen, Hun, Yi and Zhi respectively. Although they do not treat specific conditions of the Wu Shen, they can help to regulate the movements of their corresponding Shen in addition to other points chosen within a prescription.

BL-50 (Wei Cang) is on the outer branch of the Bladder channel, amongst the points mentioned above. It sits in line with the Back Shu point of the Stomach (BL-21, Wei Shu), and is sometimes considered to be more important for the Yi than BL-49 (Yi She) due to the Stomach's function of processing and digesting the thoughts that have been generated by the Yi. Stimulating BL-50 is useful for helping patients to 'digest' their thoughts and to treat obsessive thinking and pensiveness. It also helps to 'unknot' the Qi that may have been caused by worry and over-thinking.

LU-3 (Tian Fu) is classed as a Window of Heaven point. It is a point that is used to bring emotion to the surface, due to the exterior releasing nature of the Lungs, which enables the patient to acknowledge certain emotions and therefore enables them to deal with and process them. Again, due to the nature of the Lungs, it is particularly good to help patients acknowledge grief and sadness. These emotions are easily ignored by patients. This is mainly because of the effect that the emotions have on the Po and that the Po can go into a state of numbness once it becomes disturbed. Stimulating LU-3 (Tian Fu) can allow these emotions to be brought to the surface so that they can be released properly.

LU-7 (Lie Que) and **R-17 (Shan Zhong)** are both excellent points to help the patient release emotion. LU-7 helps to release emotion by bringing it to the surface and 'letting go' through the Lung channel. It is important to advise your patients that this point may provoke a reaction of crying, due to the Lungs venting excess emotion through the action of crying. R-17, on the other hand, being the Front Mu point of the Pericardium channel, releases emotion directly from the Heart. This will not necessarily evoke a reaction of crying, but could evoke the venting of emotion in the way that the corresponding emotion is likely to be released, such as shouting to vent excess anger from the Liver.

P-3 (Qu Ze) is a strong point that is useful for helping patients to 'see things more clearly' in a psychological way (not physically). This is due to its connection to both the Heart as the Heart Protector, and the Hun through its connection with the Liver Jue Yin channel. It also very useful for clearing Heat that is deep within the body.

P-4 (Xi Men) is a Xi-Cleft point, meaning that it is an excellent point for treating stagnation. Due to it being the Xi-Cleft point of the Pericardium channel, it is very good for treating stagnation that is affecting the mind and the emotions. For people who feel they are 'stuck', or for patients with depression where they feel they cannot move on, P-4 can help to resolve stagnation and allow the Shen and Hun to flow freely.

P-6 (Nei Guan) and **P-7 (Da Ling)** are both very good points for treating anxiety and palpitations by opening the chest and regulating the Heart. P-6 has a greater effect on the middle Jiao for patients who have digestive issues when they feel anxious, and also has a direct effect on spreading the Liver Qi in cases of depression due to its connection to the Liver and the Hun through Jue Yin and Blood. P-7, on the other hand, is better for patients who have Heat signs and mental restlessness when they feel anxious due to its slightly more sedating nature.

P-8 (Lao Gong) is a point located on the palm of the hand and is used to both draw Heat from the Heart and to vent excess Qi away from the chest. Think of it as an exhaust system for the Heart. It is a strong point, and very effective for those who store emotion and feel a fullness in the chest from emotions such as stress, anxiety or depression. It is also an excellent point for patients to self-massage day to day to ensure it stays open. However, it can be a relatively draining point, so it should not be used excessively when there is no excess or if there is deficiency.

DU-16 (Feng Fu), **BL-10 (Tian Zhu)** and **GB-20 (Feng Chi)** are known as the 'Gates of Consciousness', with BL-10 also being classified as a Window of Heaven point. All three points are very useful to improve the flow of Qi and Blood between the body and the brain, and help to descend Qi that becomes 'stuck' in the head. This helps to calm the mind and helps people to feel more rooted.

DU-24 (Shen Ting) is a point on the Du channel that allows the descending of Qi and the rooting of Shen due to the location of the point being on the 'tipping point' of the channel, just before it begins to descend. It is thought of like the top of a waterfall. DU-24 is a calming point used to help descend the Yang Qi once it has reached its apex (at DU-20, Bai Hui), and can be used for many types of emotion causing mental restlessness.

EX-M-HN-3 (Yin Tang) is an excellent point that is used to help calm the Shen, especially with techniques such as **Yi Zhi Chan Tui Fa**; however, it should not be used for those who experience outbursts of anger, or those who suffer from severely excess conditions such as Liver Fire or Liver Yang Rising due to it causing Qi and Blood to rise to the head and face. It is commonly used for patients with anxiety and patients who may feel nervous. It is also very good for patients where the Qi is scattered as it helps to bring people back to centre.

K-4 (Da Zhong) is a point that regulates and nourishes the Zhi through consolidating the Jing, and therefore benefits the Shen by keeping it rooted. K-4 is useful for patients who are very Yang in nature, and very cerebral where they are often in their own head a lot and overly analytical. It is also the Luo connecting point of the Kidney channel, meaning that it can be used treat the Bladder (hence its name, 'Great Goblet') for patients with low self-esteem and insecurities.

EX-N-HN-54 (An Mian) is an extra point that is literally called 'Sleep Peacefully'. It is an empirical point that can be used for any pattern that gives rise to insomnia, whether it is due to excess type or deficiency type. It is an excellent point to be used alongside DU-16 (Feng Fu) to calm and regulate the Shen.

LI-4 (He Gu) and **Lv-3 (Tai Chong)** together are known as the 'Four Gates', and help to move Qi and Blood through the channels. This helps with both pain and emotional stagnation. Whereas being used individually will help to move Qi (LI-4) and Blood (Lv-3), being used together will greatly improve the effect of resolving stagnation. This combination, however, should not be used too frequently or too carelessly, as it is a very strong combination and should not be used with patients who are too weak.

R-12 (Zhong Wan) is called 'Central Stomach', and is located on the anterior midline at the body's centre. It is a location that the Qi commonly 'knots' due to worry and over-thinking, and use of this point can greatly help to move Qi and relieve constraint due to emotion. It is a key nourishing point for the Qi at the same time as a point used to help circulate the Qi throughout the body.

R-14 (Ju Que) is the Front Mu point of the Heart, and is an excellent point to help regulate the Shen and calm the mind. It is also very good for treating anxiety by unblocking stagnation between the upper Jiao and the middle Jiao, and allowing Qi to descend from the Heart to the Kidneys to help root the Shen.

ST-25 (Tian Shu) is a key point with a vast number of functions and indication. As a great tonification (Da Bu, 大补) point, it can be used to help tonify most types of deficiency that are rooted in Qi and/or Blood. However, it is also an excellent point for bringing the mind back to centre in times of stress or anxiety, helps to focus the Yi by strengthening the Earth element (thereby helping the processing of our thoughts and actions) and harmonises the Hun and Po. It is a great all-rounder for the Shen, and is often used in many Tui Na or Acupuncture prescriptions for both mental/emotional and digestive conditions.

Anxiety

Anxiety is a broad term that can affect patients in many different ways. It is a condition that is generally categorised as a feeling of unease and often caused by an increase of stress. Patients will often find it difficult to switch off and unwind, and may show signs and symptoms such as palpitations, increased heart rate, disturbed sleep, breathing difficulties or chest oppression.

According to Chinese Medicine, anxiety primarily affects the Spleen, Lungs and Heart. It causes the Qi to become blocked in the upper part of the body, causing shortness of breath and palpitations, and prevents the Qi from descending through the diaphragm. Due to the blockage of Qi, it can also affect digestion and prevent our thoughts generated by the Yi from being processed, which gives rise to obsessive thoughts and pensiveness that subsequently affect the Spleen and Stomach.

When treating anxiety, it is very important to distinguish whether the patient is suffering from excess type Anxiety or deficiency type Anxiety. This may sound obvious to the typical Chinese Medicine practitioner, although it is not the standard way of thinking in the West. Unfortunately, most medications aimed to treat anxiety are sedatives or even hypnotics. Whereas these might be useful for patients who suffer from excess type Anxiety (such as Heart Fire type), those who suffer from deficiency type (such as Spleen Qi and Heart Blood deficiency, or Liver Blood deficiency) will likely experience no benefit or may even become worse.

To treat general anxiety conditions, the main focus should be to allow the Qi and Blood to flow freely in and out of the upper Jiao. This will allow the Qi to circulate better and the feeling of unease to diminish. Once the Qi is flowing correctly, the mind will be able to process thoughts and feelings more efficiently, and the patient will begin to feel more grounded. Once the above base sequence for regulating the Shen has been applied, perform the following sequence:

Supine position

- Begin with the patient lying face up in a relaxed supine position. Use **Ma Fa** on the face, starting at EX-M-HN-3 (Yin Tang) and wiping just above the brow to finish at EX-M-HN-9 (Tai Yang). Finish with **Rou Fa** (with the thumb) at Tai Yang. Repeat this nine times.

- Use **Ma Fa** again starting at EX-M-HN-3 (Yin Tang) and wiping upwards to finish at DU-24 (Shen Ting). Do this 36 times.

- Use **Fen Tui Fa** along the lower boarder of the clavicle, from K-27 (Shu Fu) to LU-2 (Yun Men). Repeat this for 1–2 minutes followed by **Ca Fa** with the fingers along the Ren channel for a further 1–2 minutes, between R-22 (Tian Tu) and R-14 (Ju Que) to open up the chest to release blocked Qi.

- Use **Fen Tui Fa** across the lower boarder of the rib cage, from R-14 (Ju Que) to Lv-13 (Zhang Men) to help release the diaphragm to enable a better exchange of Qi and Blood in and out of the upper Jiao.

- Finish with **Mo Fa** and **Rou Fa** on the abdomen to warm and soften the area, and allow Qi and Blood to circulate throughout the abdomen correctly.

Seated position

- Ask the patient to carefully sit up in a relaxed seated position with their arms by their side. Use **Mo Fa** on the upper back and shoulders to warm and relax the patient.

- Use **Na Fa** on the nape of the neck whilst holding their forehead to take tension out of the neck, followed by gentle **Ba Shen Fa** on the head and neck to help open up the base of the skull. Whilst performing **Na Fa**, focus on stimulating GB-20 (Feng Chi).

- Use **Gun Fa** on the upper back and shoulders, and stimulate GB-21 (Jian Jing) **An Fa** whilst the patient breathes out, to help descend Qi and drop the ribcage. Stimulate GB-21 three times.

Prone position

- Begin with **Mo Fa**, **Rou Fa** and **Gun Fa** to warm and open the back, and use a combination of **Gun Fa** and **Na Fa** on the legs to open up the leg Sinew channels. This will help to release the spine and allow Qi and Blood to regulate throughout the Du channel whilst opening the Leg channels to help root the Qi.

- Use **Nie Fa** along the Du channel in a downward direction, to help further descend the Qi. Repeat this six times.

- Use **An Fa** to stimulate BL-13 (Fei Shu), BL-15 (Xin Shu) and BL-17 (Ge Shu). Repeat this nine times, for 5–10 seconds each time.

- Finish by using **Tui Fa** to dredge down each side of the body three times, followed by pressing (**An Fa**) and holding K-1 (Yong Quan) to draw the Qi down and to root the Shen. This also helps to draw the body's awareness down to the feet and away from the head, which is an important principle when treating anxiety.

After-care advice

- Anxiety causes the Qi to become blocked in the upper Jiao, so techniques to help unblock and descend the Qi are important. Suggest that your patient stimulates K-1 (Yong Quan) with self-massage each evening to help descend the Qi and stay rooted. Deep breathing is also important, focusing on holding the outbreath for 3–4 seconds in order to stimulate Yin and release tension.

- It is important to avoid any stimulants, such as coffee, alcohol, tea or spicy foods that may raise Yang and exacerbate anxiety.

- Mindfulness techniques are useful to help regulate the Po and help the patient remain in the present to avoid anxious thoughts.

Modifications according to syndrome differentiation
The following techniques and suggestions may be added to the above routine according to the diagnosed pattern:

Spleen Qi and Heart Blood deficiency
If the Spleen Qi is deficient and the Heart Blood has been consumed, which may manifest as a tendency to worry or over-think, palpitations, insomnia, low appetite or loose stools, add the following:

- Stimulate ST-25 (Tian Shu) with **Rou Fa** or **Yi Zhi Chan Tui Fa** to help nourish the Yi and Blood by tonifying the Ying Qi.

- Use **Rou Fa** on the lower abdomen to promote the movement of Qi within the middle Jiao and improve the production of Qi and Blood.

- Use **Gun Fa** and **Rou Fa** on the back, focusing on BL-15 (Xin Shu) and BL-20 (Pi Shu) to strengthen the Heart and Spleen respectively, and help the circulation of Qi within the upper and middle Jiao.

Phlegm misting the mind (Phlegm harassing the Heart)
If there is anxiety caused by Phlegm misting the mind, which may manifest as lethargy, mental confusion and depression, insomnia, a rattle in the throat or a thick, sticky tongue coating, add the following:

- Stimulate ST-40 (Feng Long) with **Yi Zhi Chan Tui Fa** or **An Fa** to transform and move Phlegm.

- Use **Rou Fa** along the Pericardium channel, focusing on P-4 (Xi Men) and P-5 (Jian Shi) to help transform Phlegm and regulate the Heart Shen.

Heart and Kidney Yin deficiency

If there is anxiety caused by a Heart and Kidney disharmony leading to deficiency of the Heart and Kidney Yin, manifesting as palpitations, insomnia, poor memory, tinnitus, lower back pain, night sweating or anxiety that is worse in the evening, add the following:

- Stimulate K-4 (Da Zhong) and K-6 (Zhang Hai) with **Rou Fa** to nourish the Kidneys and ascend the Yin Fluids to the Heart.

- Use **Tui Fa** with the thumb from R-17 (Shan Zhong) to R-14 (Ju Que). This helps to clear Heat from the Heart that may have arisen from the deficiency of Yin, and works on opening the Ren Mai (known as the 'Sea of Yin'). Repeat this nine times.

- Use **Rou Fa** and **Gun Fa** on the back, working from BL-14 (Jue Yin Shu) to BL-23 (Shen Shu) for 4–5 minutes.

- Due to the nature of Yin, it is very important to work on the patient's diet when treating Yin conditions, as Tui Na alone will struggle to nourish Yin without the addition of substances such as food or herbs. It is important that the patient's diet consists of moistening foods in addition to limiting foods that are too warming or drying. It is also important that the patient stays well hydrated, and avoids any stimulants such as coffee and cocoa.

Heart Fire

If there is anxiety caused by Heart Fire, which may manifest as palpitations, feeling of Heat and excessive thirst, mental restlessness, insomnia with dream-disturbed sleep, tongue ulcers or talking quickly and excessively, add the following:

- To open up the Heart and Pericardium channels, use **Rou Fa** along the Heart channel from HT-3 (Shao Hai) to HT-7 (Shen Men) six times, followed by stimulating P-8 (Lao Gong) and EX-UE-8 (Wai Lao Gong) simultaneously for 1–2 minutes using **Rou Fa** with the thumb.

- Use **Tui Fa** from R-14 (Ju Que) to the navel (R-8, Shen Que) for 1–2 minutes to descend the Qi and drain Fire.

- Use **Gun Fa** on the back, travelling from BL-15 (Xin Shu) to BL-18 (Gan Shu) for 3–5 minutes to regulate the Heart and Liver.

Liver Qi stagnation

If there is anxiety due to Liver Qi stagnation restricting the flow of Qi and Blood within the chest, manifesting as a fullness or discomfort in the chest, plum stone throat, irritability, sighing or a taut pulse, add the following:

- With certain types of anxiety that involve Liver Qi stagnation, Qi can often become blocked around the base of the throat. This is known as Plum Stone Qi (Mei He Qi, 梅核氣). If this is present, stimulate R-22 (Tian Tu) with **Yi Zhi Chan Tui Fa** to unblock the Qi and resolve local stagnation.

- With the patient in a seated position, use **Cuo Fa** on the intercostals to improve the flow of Liver Qi.

- Stimulate P-6 (Nei Guan) and Lv-3 (Tai Chong) with **An Fa** or **Rou Fa** to improve the circulation of Qi in the chest and to help the Liver's function of governing the free flow of Qi as part of the Jue Yin channel.

Lung Qi deficiency

If there is anxiety due to a deficiency of the Lung Qi causing a lack of regulation of the Heart rate and circulation within the chest, which may manifest as shortness of breath, a disliking of talking or a soft voice, fatigue, weak cough or panic attacks accompanied by palpitations and shallow breathing, or a feeling of sadness and melancholy, add the following:

- Gently use **Gun Fa** and **Rou Fa** on the upper and mid back, placing emphasis on BL-13 (Fei Shu), BL-17 (Ge Shu), and BL-20 (Pi Shu) to direct Yang Qi to the Lungs, release the diaphragm and promote the acquired Qi (to strengthen the Lungs) respectively.

- Use **Yao Fa** and **Ba Shen Fa** on the shoulders and arms to help open up the chest and the Lung Sinew channel. Stretch open the chest by pulling back on the shoulders and performing **Ba Shen Fa** on the neck and head.

- Use **An Fa** or **Rou Fa** to stimulate LU-9 (Tai Yuan) to direct the Yuan Qi to the Lungs.

Depression

Depression is a complex emotion, and a term used very broadly in the Western sense. It can really be due to any combination of channel or organ dysfunction. It is important to clarify what type of depression the patient is suffering from by understanding key aspects of how the condition is affecting the patient, how the patient is reacting to the feeling of depression and how the depression was caused in the first place.

Ultimately, depression is always due to a stagnation of Qi, with the main type of depression in Chinese being called Yu (鬱, stagnation) Zheng (症, disease). One of the key characteristics of all types of depression is a feeling of being trapped and unable to move forward in life. As the Hun likes to move and wander freely without being restricted or supressed, this stagnation primarily affects the Hun (and therefore the Liver), and its relationship with the other Shen (mainly the Po due to the Metal/Wood relationship through the controlling cycle, and the Shen due to the Liver/Heart relationship through the Blood).

Stagnation and constraint

Depression is always rooted in *stagnation*, and will therefore always present with patterns of a *constraint within the Hun*. Due to the controlling and restraining relationship of the *Hun* and *Po,* the focus in treatment of depression is often placed on relieving constraint of the Hun that is caused by the over-control of the Po.

Depending on the patient's signs and symptoms, and the way that they cope and react to depression, we can determine which emotions and aspects of the mind are being affected by taking the following into account:

- **Hun type:** If the patient is reacting to situations in an irritable fashion and having feelings of frustration and anger, it indicates that the patient's depression has its roots in the dysfunction of the Liver and therefore the Hun. This may have arisen from stress and overwork, particularly due to work-related situations.

- **Shen type:** If the patient has accompanying sadness, lack of joy, and if the patient's depression arose due to a situation of heartbreak, this indicates that the patient's Heart and therefore Shen may be disturbed.

- **Po type:** If the patient is showing signs of numbness yet a feeling of hopelessness, this will indicate that the Po and Lungs are involved, which are likely to be over-controlling on the Hun (via the Metal/Wood controlling cycle). Patients with this type of depression may also act withdrawn and isolate themselves from society. This type of depression often arises from a situation of grief or loss, such as the loss of a family member, a loved one or the loss of sense of self.

- **Zhi type:** If the patient lacks motivation or drive, such as having little or no willpower to put mechanisms into place to recover from depression, this may indicate that the Kidneys are involved and therefore the Zhi. Patients with this type of depression may also find themselves experiencing 'bad luck' and feel that nothing is going right for them as they may have lost their connection to their life path.

- **Yi type:** If the patient is experiencing rumination, an inability to switch off, and continues to think obsessively about things, it may indicate that the Stomach and Spleen (and therefore the Yi) are involved. The Qi will begin to 'knot' in the middle Jiao, most commonly around R-12 (Zhong Wan), and patients may experience digestive difficulties with their emotional state likely to be affected by a poor diet.

When treating patients with depression, perform the following routine in addition to implementing the modifications depending on the type of depression (or combination of types) found below:

Supine position

- As all types of depression have an element of Qi stagnation, begin by using **Ba Shen Fa** on each major joint to open the Qi Men and allow the tendons and sinews to stretch. This should be performed in a gentle and relaxing manner, and helps the Qi to flow freely.

- Use **An Fa** or **Rou Fa** to stimulate the Lung and Pericardium Xi-Cleft points (LU-6, Kong Zui and P-4, Xi Men) to help purge stored emotions within the body.

- Use **Yi Zhi Chan Tui Fa** or **Rou Fa** on DU-24 (Shen Ting) to open the Du channel and direct any stagnant Qi downwards and out of the head.

Seated position

- Use **Cuo Fa** on the intercostals to improve the flow of Liver Qi, and to help movement of the Hun by stimulating both the Liver and Gall Bladder channels.

- Use **Yao Fa** and **Ba Shen Fa** on the head and neck to lift the Qi and allow Yang Qi to flow freely up the Du channel and enter the Brain. Doing this also helps to encourage a better upright posture, which in turn can help the flow of Qi through the Bladder channel and improve the patient's self-esteem and self-worth due to the energetic function of the Bladder channel.

Prone position

- Begin with releasing tension from the shoulders and neck with **Na Fa**, and using **An Fa** or **Rou Fa** to strongly stimulate GB-20 (Feng Chi) and DU-16 (Feng Fu). Use **Gun Fa** and **Rou Fa** on the back to help relax the patient and encourage the flow of Qi and Blood through the Bladder channel. Focus on the Shen points located on the outer Bladder channel, depending on which of the Shen requires harmonising.

- Use **Nie Fa** along the spine in an upward direction to activate the Du channel and help to raise Yang Qi to the head and support the Brain.

- Finish by using **Tui Fa** to dredge down each side of the body three times, followed by pressing (using **An Fa**) and holding K-1 (Yong Quan) to draw the Qi down and to root the Shen.

After-care advice

- Suggest to the patient that they set goals for themselves so that they can see a way forward to move out of stagnation. The Hun like achievement and ambition. Suggest that the goals are achievable so that the reward system of the mind is stimulated. This helps to harmonise the Hun and the Po.

- Avoid stagnating foods and eating habits. Heavy foods such as meat should be reduced (but not avoided), so that the Qi can rise and circulate properly. Time should be taken whilst eating, and eating should be done at times when the mind is calm and void of any excessive emotion.

- Gentle exercise and stretching is important to encourage movement of the Liver Qi and to again avoid stagnation.

Modifications according to the Wu Shen (Five Spirits)

The following techniques and suggestions have been made according to the different types of depression based on the involvement of the Wu Shen rather than the usual Zang Fu syndrome differentiation, as found elsewhere in the book. It is essential when treating mental/emotional conditions that we are familiar with the different characteristics, functions and dysfunctions on the Wu Shen.

Hun type depression

- Use **Gun Fa** on the back, focusing on and stimulating BL-18 (Gan Shu) and BL-47 (Hun Men), and use a combination of **Gun Fa** and **Rou Fa** along the Liver and Kidney Sinew channels.

- Stimulate Lv-3 (Tai Chong) using **An Fa**, **Rou Fa** or **Yi Zhi Chan Tui Fa** to nourish the Liver Blood and stimulate the free flow of Qi.

- Use **Cuo Fa** on the ribs to release tension in the hypochondrial regions and to 'soften' the Liver.

- It is important that the patient stretches and moves regularly in order to help the Liver and stimulate the Hun.

Shen type depression

- Use **Gun Fa** on the back, focusing on and stimulating BL-15 (Xin Shu) and BL-44 (Shen Tang), and use a combination of **Tui Fa**, **Na Fa** and **Rou Fa** along the Heart and Pericardium Sinew channels.

- Stimulate P-7 (Da Ling) using **An Fa**, **Rou Fa** or **Yi Zhi Chan Tui Fa**.

- Use **Ca Fa** on the sternum to open the chest cavity and stimulate Qi flow around the Heart.

- It is important that the patient finds a way to express themselves, such as dancing, painting, writing and so on. whilst also stilling the mind in order to strengthen the Heart.

Po type depression

- Use **Gun Fa** on the back, focusing on and stimulating BL-13 (Fei Shu) and BL-42 (Po Hu), and use a combination of **Tui Fa**, **Na Fa** and **Rou Fa** along the Lung and Large Intestine Sinew channels.

- Stimulate LU-3 (Tian Fu) using **An Fa**, **Rou Fa** or **Yi Zhi Chan Tui Fa** to assist in the processing of grief.

- Use **Fen Tui Fa** across the lower boarder of the rib cage, from R-14 (Ju Que) to Lv-13 (Zhang Men), to help release the diaphragm to enable a better exchange of Qi and Blood in and out of the upper Jiao.

- Techniques that help to regulate the breath are important to strengthen the Lungs and stimulate the Po.

Zhi type depression

- Use **Gun Fa** on the back, focusing on and stimulating BL-23 (Shen Shu) and BL-52 (Zhi Shi), and use a combination of **Gun Fa** and **Rou Fa** along the Kidney Sinew channel.

- Stimulate K-4 (Da Zhong) using **An Fa**, **Rou Fa** or **Yi Zhi Chan Tui Fa** to nourish the Zhi and root the Shen.

- Use **Mo Fa** and **Ca Fa** to warm and regulate the lower back, focusing on DU-4 (Ming Men) to stimulate the motivation and drive of the Zhi.

- It is important that the patient feels rooted in life and has a support network in place in order to strengthen the Kidneys and nourish the Zhi.

Yi type depression

- Use **Gun Fa** on the back, focusing on and stimulating BL-20 (Pi Shu) and BL-45 (Yi Xi), and use a combination of **Gun Fa** and **Rou Fa** along the leg aspects of the Spleen and Stomach Sinew channels.

- Stimulate SP-3 (Tai Bai) using **An Fa**, **Rou Fa** or **Yi Zhi Chan Tui Fa** to strengthen the functions of the Spleen and nourish the Yi.

- Use **Mo Fa** and **Rou Fa** on the abdomen (focusing around R-12) to warm and soften the area. This allows the Qi and Blood to circulate throughout the abdomen correctly, to assist in digestion and the processing of thoughts.

- Diet is important to help regulate the Spleen and the Yi. This should be advised according to the patient's individual constitution.

Complex type depression

More often than not, *depression* will be a *combination* of the above types, so it may be necessary to *combine treatment methods*.

Chapter 12

Respiratory Disorders

When treating respiratory disorders, we understandably focus much of our treatment on the Lung system and its associated channels. Although other organs and channels are expected to be involved, such as the Kidneys for their assistance in grasping the Lung Qi and the Liver for its assistance in circulating the Qi, treatment of the Lungs and the chest cavity is essential for successful treatment of any respiratory condition. In addition to the Lungs, however, it is almost always necessary to work with the Diaphragm in order for it to allow correct movement of Qi throughout the torso. This means that we may need to work on a number of Sinew channels, as quite a few of them attach on to various parts of the diaphragm. Although energetically it is the Lungs that are said to control respiration and regulate the Qi through breath, it is the diaphragm that helps to control and regulate the breath physically. Unless the diaphragm is moving freely, respiration will not be smooth or deep enough, and the Lungs will not be able to carry out their function effectively.

The delicate organ

According to Chinese Medicine theory, the Lungs are a 'delicate' organ, and should therefore be treated carefully in as much as treatment should not be too powerful or too drastic. When patients present with Lung syndromes, especially of deficiency type, it is relatively easy to exacerbate symptoms by agitating the Lungs from a treatment that is too strong. For example, with a strong treatment, it is possible to stimulate the Lungs in a way that causes the channels to constrict and bring on a tight chest and wheezing. This should be avoided by treating gently. *Less is more in regards to treating the Lungs.*

Unlike many of the internal organs, the Lungs can be affected by both internal and external diseases. This is because the Lungs are essentially the most external of the internal organs, and are therefore vulnerable to external conditions such as the common cold, allergies or the flu. Certain Tui Na techniques can be used to help the Lungs to release the exterior (using the sweating therapeutic method), allowing external pathogenic factors that are causing conditions such as the common cold and the flu to be expelled. In addition to this, Cupping therapy was classically used to draw out external pathogens and to allow the Lungs to expel them through the pores of the skin. Cupping therapy is an excellent adjunct to Tui Na for the treatment of respiratory conditions for this reason.

Apart from external factors, such as the common cold or the flu, most respiratory conditions are due to three main reasons: weakness of the Lungs, dysfunction of the diaphragm or emotional stress.

Weakness of the Lungs may or may not be due to congenital factors. One of the primary functions of the Lungs is to receive Qi by breathing in Air, and transforming this into a type of refined Qi that can be used within the body. The more efficient the Lungs are, the better the refinement of Qi (equally, the cleaner the Air, the less work the Lungs need to do, and the stronger they will become). If the Lungs are weak for whatever reason, they will struggle to both effectively refine and descend the Qi, which is one of their key functions. If the Qi is not refined enough, this will lead to shallow breathing and shortness of breath as the body tries to pull in more Air to increase the amount of refined Qi within the body. If the Qi is not descending properly, this will again lead to shallow breathing, and cause both coughing and wheezing. Lastly, external factors may invade the body because the Lungs are too weak to regulate the exterior. This will cause the patient to have a weak immune system and be prone to coughs and colds.

The second factor is due to dysfunction of the diaphragm. As mentioned previously, it is the diaphragm that helps to both regulate the breath and physically assist the Lungs to carry out their function of receiving the Qi and circulating Qi and Body Fluids throughout the body. When the diaphragm becomes dysfunctional, by becoming stuck or weak, for instance, the breathing will be shallow and laboured. This prevents the Lungs from taking sufficiently deep breaths, and creates a lack of power to disseminate the Qi and Body Fluids throughout the body. This will lead to stagnation and eventually to the weakness of the Lungs. A dysfunctional diaphragm will also inhibit the exchange of Qi between the three Jiaos by preventing the transfer of Qi between the Lungs, Spleen and Kidneys. This will cause the Lung Qi to ascend, giving rise to coughing, wheezing and shortness of breath.

The third key factor to cause respiratory conditions is emotional stress, especially that which is caused by grief. Emotions are essentially pathogens that arise from the interactions between different aspects of the mind in response to both internal and external stimuli, and it is up to the Lungs to help to release and let go of them. If there is (for whatever reason) a lot of emotion to deal with, the Lungs become overwhelmed and therefore unable to let go and release emotion. This causes tension and stagnation within both the Lungs and the diaphragm, and can, over time, cause weakness and dysfunction of the Lungs. In these instances, identifying the emotion and enabling the processing of the emotion are important and necessary for successful treatment of the respiratory condition. Emotional disorders have been discussed earlier in this section.

When diagnosing respiratory conditions, in addition to assessing the diaphragm, we need to pay attention to other signs and symptoms. It is essential that we listen to the breathing and also to the cough if coughing is a symptom. We also need to inquire about the type of cough and the quality of any phlegm that is being coughed up if any. For instance, if the patient is breathing very softly and feebly, it will indicate a deficiency type syndrome, whereas if the patient is breathing heavily and audibly, it will likely indicate an excess type syndrome. In regards to the cough, we need to distinguish if it is weak (deficiency), strong (excess), dry (Dryness) or loose and productive (Dampness or Phlegm). We also need to know about the colour and quality of any Phlegm that is produced, such as watery or white (Cold), or yellow and thick (Heat). In summary, diagnosis is key with treatment variation.

Key acupressure points

Although it is important to choose acupressure points according to their functions and indications in respect to your Chinese Medicine differential diagnosis, the following points are just a few that are especially beneficial to help with respiratory conditions.

EX-M-BW-1 (Ding Chuan) is an extra point located at the top of the back that helps to alleviate wheezing, hence its name Ding Chuan (meaning to 'Calm Wheezing'). It has been found to help with coughing and wheezing, and is also good during an acute asthma attack to help calm the Lungs.

LU-1 (Zhong Fu) is the Front Mu point of the Lungs, and is therefore tender when there is a Lung pathology. It is an excellent point for opening the chest to give space for the Lungs to breathe fully, and helps the Lungs function of descending the Qi. It is also this point that the Lung channel merges with the Spleen channel to create Tai Yin, which is why it is good to strengthen the immune system when patients are prone to the common cold or the flu.

LU-3 (Tian Fu) is classed as a Window of Heaven point, and helps to release the chest that is tight due to emotion, in particular, grief. As a Window of Heaven point, it also enables the patient to recognise their emotional state and allow the processing of their particular emotions. This is especially useful for patients who appear emotionally numb.

LU-7 (Lie Que) helps to guide Qi to the Lungs in addition to helping the Lungs disperse fluids and release the exterior. Using this point to release the exterior helps to both expel pathogens from and emotions that are stored at the Wei level.

LU-9 (Tai Yuan) is the Yuan-Source point of the Lung channel and helps to direct Yuan Qi to the Lungs in order to strengthen them. Yuan-Source points are often used to directly treat and regulate their corresponding organ, especially any kind of imbalance within them. LU-9 is indicated for Lung deficiency and also for eliminating pathogenic factors within the Lungs by strengthening the Wei Qi and the anti-pathogenic (Zheng) Qi.

LU-5 (Che Zi) and **LU-10 (Yu Ji)** are both cooling points for the Lung system. LU-5 is a He-Sea point, and is used to reduce Heat from the Lung organs themselves, with signs such as a dry cough or coughing up yellow phlegm. It is a very good point for internal Heat within the Lungs. LU-10, on the other hand, is more for external Heat. It is a Ying-Spring point, which is classically indicated for any kind of Heat pathogen within the channel. LU-10, being the Ying-Spring point on the Lung channel, also helps to clear Heat from the throat and the air passages in addition to drawing out any Heat from within the channel itself, such as inflammation.

R-22 (Tian Tu) is located at the base of the neck, in the centre of the suprasternal fossa. This is the region of the body where we can suffer from emotional stagnation just before we are able to process it and let go. Therefore, using this point can help people express emotion and unblock any stagnation that it may have caused. R-22 is also an excellent point to supress a cough and unblock any stagnation that has been caused by wrongfully ascending Qi.

ST-13 (Qi Hu) helps to move Qi from the head region and into the chest region. This is why it is known as 'Qi Hu', meaning Qi Doorway. ST-13 is an excellent point to nourish the Lungs and open the chest to allow Qi to flow within the upper body. It is also an excellent point to supress a cough.

K-1 (Yong Quan) is the lowest point on the body, positioned on the sole of the foot, and helps to draw down the Lung Qi to help calm wheezing, especially during an asthma attack. It is a sedating point, so it should not be used too much, and it should also not be stimulated in times of deficiency. However, during times when the Qi is unable to descend, such as when experiencing an asthma attack or intense coughing, K-1 can be very useful in calming the Qi and drawing it downwards.

K-27 (Shu Fu) is a local point located on the chest just below the clavicle, and is an excellent point to descend the Qi by activating the Kidney channel (which functions to ground and descend the Qi). In addition to descending the Qi, which helps the Lungs to self-regulate, K-27 also transforms Phlegm and helps to supress a cough that has been caused by the ascending of Lung Qi.

Back Shu points of the Lung (BL-13, Fei Shu) and Diaphragm (BL-17, Ge Shu) are useful for treating all types of respiratory disorders. Other Back Shu points should also be taken into account depending on the differential diagnosis. For instance, the Kidney Shu point (BL-23, Shen Shu) is important for conditions where the Kidneys are not grasping the Lung Qi, as all Back Shu points help to release Heat from their corresponding organ in addition to transporting Yang Qi from the Du channel to the corresponding organ in order to treat deficiency conditions.

Releasing the diaphragm

First of all, we must assess the patient's breathing and diaphragm, as discussed in Section 2. It is important to assess the breathing and engagement of the diaphragm in any respiratory condition, as incorrect breathing by the patient will prevent any treatment from being entirely effective. To release the diaphragm:

- Begin with asking the patient to lie on their back in a relaxed supine position, and perform **Fen Tui Fa** on their chest beneath the clavicle, stimulating K-27 (Shu Fu), ST-13 (Qi Hu) and LU-2 (Yun Men) to help open the chest and descend the Qi. In this position, also use **Tui Fa** on the region of GB-21 (Jian Jing) bi-laterally to help descend the ribcage and release tension from the shoulders.

- Using **Rou Fa** (with the thumbs), stimulate the meeting point of the three Arm Yin Sinew channels. This is to help release and activate the aspect of the Diaphragm that connects to the three Arm Yin channels.

- Use **Ba Shen Fa** on each leg to gently decompress the hip joints and to help release and activate the three Sinew channels, and follow by using **Ya Fa** or **An Fa** to stimulate the meeting point of the three Leg Yin sinews at the lower abdomen. This, like the above, is to help release the aspect of the Diaphragm that connects to the three Leg Yin channels.

- Next, ask the patient to lie in a relaxed position on their side. Gently place your palms onto their ribs, and hook your fingers underneath their ribs to touch the diaphragm at around the area of the Liver/Gall Bladder channels. *Be cautious to not go in too hard, as this can hurt the Liver and Spleen. If there is tension in the external muscles groups preventing you from hooking under the ribs, ask the patient to bring their knees up slightly to help release any tension within the abdomen.*

- As the patient breathes in, push your fingers into the diaphragm and gently rub the underside of the ribs. As the patient breathes out, gently shake and vibrate your hands to help further release the diaphragm. Repeat this for three to five breaths, with the patient lying on each side. It is important to note here that we are *not* lifting or pulling on the ribs. We are simply hooking our fingers underneath and behind the ribs so that we can touch the diaphragm.

- After releasing both sides, ask the patient to take a seated position. From behind, reach around the patient and hook your fingers again underneath their ribs, starting in the region of the ST channel (it is important to avoid the centre, as this is where the solar plexus is located). Ask the patient to take a deep breath and to fold at the waist as they breathe out – this allows you to get deeper into the abdomen with your fingers as it begins to relax. When your fingers are touching the diaphragm at the end of the breath, shake them from side to side gently to help relax the tissues.

- Ask the patient to lie on their front in prone position. Use **Rou Fa** and **Tui Fa** along the paraspinal muscles of the thoracic spine, and focus on stimulating BL-17 (Ge Shu). *Sometimes the diaphragm may be stuck due to restriction of the thoracic spine.* Ensure that the spine is mobilised and moving properly. This can be done using simple Tui Na techniques, or may require **An Ya Fu Wei Fa** or **Ban Fa**.

- Finally, ask the patient to turn over again onto their back in a relaxed supine position, and use **An Fa** to strongly press K-1 (Yong Quan) for 2–3 minutes whilst the patient breathes slowly, deeply and calmly. It is important here that the patient remains in a 'Yin' state, so a Yin breathing pattern is preferred, such as breathing in for 4–5 seconds, immediately breathing out for 4–5 seconds, and holding the breath *out* for 4–5 seconds before repeating again.

- Once the diaphragm has been released, it is important to work again on the muscles of the chest and anterior aspect of the neck. This is because chest breathing can often cause shortening of these Sinew channels in the upper chest and neck area, which pull upwards on the diaphragm. It is important to relax these to help posture and ensure the diaphragm does not become stuck again.

Treatment of conditions affecting the respiratory system

To treat general respiratory conditions, the main focus should be to strengthen the Lung Qi and open the chest cavity to allow the flow of Qi in and out of the chest, and to relieve any chest fullness. This will allow the Lungs to become stronger if deficient, and/or expel any pathogenic factors that may be present. Once the above sequence for releasing the diaphragm has been applied, perform the following sequence:

Supine position

- Begin with gentle **Ba Shen Fa** and **Dou Fa** on the upper limbs to open up the shoulders and allow Qi to flow through the Lung channels.

- Use **Rou Fa** with the thumb to stimulate R-22 (Tian Tu) for 1 minute, followed by **Fen Tui Fa** below the clavicle passing through K-27 (Shu Fu), ST-13 (Qi Hu), and ending at LU-1 (Zhong Fu).

- Push using **Tui Fa** from R-17 (Shan Zhong) to the navel (R-8, Shen Que) to help descend the Zong Qi from the Lungs to the Kidneys.

- Use **An Fa** to strongly stimulate GB-21 (Jian Jing) to descend the Qi and drop the ribcage by releasing tension from the shoulders.

Seated position

- Use **Cuo Fa** on the intercostal to help free the ribs and release any tension.

- Perform **Pai Fa** and **Ji Fa** to the upper back to release any Phlegm obstruction within the Lungs.

Prone position

- Begin with **Mo Fa** and **Rou Fa** to open the channels on the back and relax the patient.

- Use **Fen Tui Fa** on the upper back, focusing on the levels of T3 (BL-13, Fei Shu) and T7 (BL-17, Ge Shu).

- Use **Tui Fa** to push down the back to assist in the descending of Qi. Do this three times each side.

- Use **An Fa** to stimulate EX-M-BW-1 (Ding Chuan), BL-13 (Fei Shu), BL-17 (Ge Shu) and BL-23 (Shen Shu).

- Use **Gun Fa** and **Rou Fa** along the Bladder Sinew channel of the back to help open and release the ribs.

- Use **Ji Fa** to break up any stagnation within the Lungs, then **Pai Fa** to disperse Qi within the channels.

- Finish with the dredging action of **Tui Fa** with the 'Tiger's Mouth' from the upper back down to the ankles to dredge the channels and to direct Qi downwards. Do this three times each side, then use **An Fa** for 1 minute on K-1 (Yong Quan) to again ground the Qi.

After-care advice

- Certain respiratory conditions can cause a lot of emotion and stress. Asthma attacks, for instance, can be a scary thing – it's not nice to suddenly feel like you cannot breathe! Although it is difficult in some cases, it is important that the patient knows not to panic. Once panic sets in, the Kidneys find it even more difficult to grasp the Lung Qi and the Liver causes tension throughout the whole body, making the airways even more constricted. Learning to stay relaxed during an asthma attack can make a huge difference. More often than not, due to the scary nature of an asthma attack, patients will also forget to breathe out fully as they concentrate so much on getting the breath in. This prevents them from taking in enough air and again draws the Qi upwards as they become more Yang. Encourage patients to fully breathe out and relax their diaphragm as much as possible.

- Self-massage at LU-1 (Zhong Fu), using **Rou Fa** with the fingers, followed by stretching open the Lu channel and pulling on the thumb can help a great deal to open the airways and allow the Lung Qi to flow freely and strongly through the Lung channel. This can help to nourish the Lung Qi in addition to releasing external pathogens.

- The Lungs do not like lying down, so it can be useful to use an extra pillow whilst sleeping during acute flare-ups of any respiratory condition. If it is uncomfortable to sleep with an extra pillow, suggest lying on the side as this will take pressure away from the throat.

Modifications according to syndrome differentiation

The following techniques and suggestions may be added to the above routine according to the diagnosed pattern.

Lung deficiency

If there is a deficiency of the Lungs, which may manifest as feeble breathing, a disliking of talking or a weak cough, add the following:

- Stimulate LU-1 (Zhong Fu) and ST-36 (Zu San Li) using **An Fa, Rou Fa** or **Yi Zhi Chan Tui Fa.**

- Ask the patient to gently take a deep breath, and hold their breath in for 3–5 seconds whilst stimulating LU-9 (Tai Yuan) using **An Fa** or **Rou Fa** with the thumb. Repeat this for nine breaths.

Kidney deficiency not grasping the Lung Qi

If the Kidneys are deficient and failing to grasp the Lung Qi, which may manifest as breathing in the chest only, feeble breathing or possible lower back pain, add the following:

- Stimulate R-4 (Guan Yuan), LU-7 (Lie Que) and K-3 (Tai Xi) using **An Fa, Rou Fa** or **Yi Zhi Chan Tui Fa.**

- Ask the patient to gently take a deep breath, then breathe out fully yet comfortably and hold their breath out for 3–5 seconds whilst stimulating K-1 (Yong Quan) using **An Fa** or **Rou Fa** with the thumb. Repeat this for nine breaths.

- Use **Ca Fa** on both sides of the spine from BL-13 (Fei Shu) to BL-23 (Shen Shu).

Spleen and Lung deficiency

If the Spleen and Lungs are both deficient, manifesting as feeble breathing, shortness of breath with a weak cough, or a disliking of talking accompanied with a low appetite, poor digestion or loose stools, add the following:

- Stimulate SP-3 (Tai Bai), R-6 (Qi Hai) and LU-9 (Tai Yuan) using **An Fa, Rou Fa** or **Yi Zhi Chan Tui Fa.**

- Perform **Ca Fa** across the abdomen for 2–3 minutes to create a gentle warmth in the middle Jiao.

Dryness impairing the Lungs

If the Lungs are impaired by Dryness or a lack of moisture, manifesting as a dry mouth and nasal passages with a dry, raspy cough, add the following:

- Stimulate LU-7 (Lie Que) and K-6 (Zhao Hai) using **An Fa, Rou Fa** or **Yi Zhi Chan Tui Fa.**

- Diet is important to help generate fluids within the body, and it is essential that the patient is drinking sufficient fluids. Milk is a very useful substance to help clean and lubricate the Lungs. This should, however, be kept to a small amount each day, and goat's milk is preferred.

Phlegm obstructing the Lungs

If the Lungs are obstructed by Phlegm, which may manifest as a productive and loose cough in addition to a thick tongue coating, add the following:

- Stimulate ST-36 (Zu San Li), ST-40 (Feng Long) and P-6 (Nei Guan) using **An Fa**, **Rou Fa** or **Yi Zhi Chan Tui Fa**.

- Press firmly on LU-2 (Yun Men) with **An Fa** whilst asking the patient to cough. Repeat this six times to help dislodge any Phlegm stagnation.

- The patient should be advised to avoid any greasy foods in addition to any dairy products such as milk or yoghurt.

Wind Heat invading the Lungs

If the patient is suffering from Wind Heat invading the Lungs, which will manifest as slight fever and aversion to Heat, sore throat, blocked nose with thick yellow mucous and a loud cough, add the following:

- Use **Ca Fa** along the Bladder Sinew channel (most exterior channel) and Du channel to cause the sweating method.

- Stimulate LU-10 (Yu Ji), SJ-5 (Wai Guan) and LI-11 (Qu Chi) using **An Fa**, **Rou Fa** or **Yi Zhi Chan Tui Fa**.

Wind Cold invading the Lungs

If the patient is suffering from Wind Cold invading the Lungs, which will manifest as chills with aversion to Cold, runny nose and sneezing, headache with soreness of the neck and lower back, add the following:

- Use **Ca Fa** along the Bladder Sinew channel (most exterior channel) and Du channel to cause the sweating method.

- Stimulate BL-12 (Feng Men) and DU-14 (Da Zhui) using **An Fa, Rou Fa** or **Yi Zhi Chan Tui Fa**.

- If headaches occur in the occiput (Tai Yang headaches), stimulate BL-10 (Tian Zhu) and SI-3 (Hou Xi). If headaches occur in the frontal region (Yang Ming headaches), stimulate GB-14 (Yang Bai), EX-M-HN-1 (Yin Yang) and ST-8 (Tou Wei). If headaches occur at the temple region (Shao Yang headaches), stimulate GB-8 (Shuai Gu) and EX-M-HN-9 (Tai Yang).

Chapter 13

Digestive Disorders

When treating digestive disorders, we are primarily treating disorders of the Spleen, Stomach and/or Intestines directly or indirectly. Of course other organs assist in digestion, such as the Kidneys and Heart, which help provide the Spleen with the heat necessary for digestion, and the Liver and Gall Bladder provide the ability to keep things moving freely, although all digestive disorders ultimately come down to the main digestive organs, naturally. This is because it is the Stomach and Spleen that essentially drive the digestive function, with the intestines playing a secondary role in absorbing and transforming the pure and nutritious substances, whilst excreting the impure waste products.

Most digestive disorders are due to two factors – the first being diet. In addition to treating patients with Tui Na for their digestive disorders, it is essential that their diet is looked at and advice is given to help alter their diet to suit their constitutional needs in addition to rectifying their issues. Advice on eating habits (such as to avoid eating whilst on the go, when stressed or with poor posture) is equally as important as the food that is eaten when treating digestive disorders, especially when the disorders are emotionally orientated. *Healing with Whole Foods* by Paul Pitchford and (the less heavy) *Chinese System of Natural Cures* by Henry C. Lu are particularly good books to use for information relating to general Chinese food therapy.

The second factor that is a major cause of digestive disorders is stress and emotion. From a Chinese Medicine perspective, it is considered to be the Liver that ensures our emotions flow freely and are vented sufficiently. If the Liver is unable to do this (perhaps due to overwhelming stress or a current lifestyle situation), it begins to feel constrained and we suffer from what is called Qi stagnation. The digestive system is heavily reliant on our Qi flowing freely and as it should in order to aid with the processing of foods and transportation throughout the digestive system. When the Liver Qi stagnates and emotions are not resolved, it begins to affect the digestive system first and foremost. This is because the abdomen is considered to be the repository of all unresolved and stored emotion. Although it is the Zang organs that give rise to and/or are affected by specific emotions primarily, it is the Fu organs (that is, the bowels) that help to process and regulate the emotions (more about this has been explained previously, in Chapter 11, on emotional disorders). By ensuring that the Qi is flowing smoothly through the channels and through the abdomen where the Fu organs are situated, the body can sufficiently process emotion allowing for a smoother flow of Qi, Blood and Body Fluids throughout the abdomen. As a result, this alleviates many digestive disorders such as inflammation, constipation, bloating, diarrhoea and so on.

Key acupressure points

Although it is important to choose acupressure points according to their functions and indications in respect to your Chinese Medicine differential diagnosis, the following points are just a few that are especially regarded for their use to regulate the digestive system.

ST-25 (Tian Shu) is known as one of the great tonification (Da Bu, 大补) points of the body, and is considered to be one of the most important points for digestive disorders of both excess and deficient type due to its harmonising nature. It is also the Front Mu point of the Large Intestine, making it a key point for any condition involving the intestine such as constipation or diarrhoea.

Lv-13 (Zhang Men) is the Front Mu point of the Spleen, essentially making it the Spleen point on the Liver channel – this is an excellent point for treating disorders of the Spleen that are caused by excess conditions of the Liver (such as irritable bowel syndrome, IBS, caused by stress and emotional irritation). Some schools of thought within Chinese Medicine believe that the Liver should be treated in any disorder of the digestive system due to its influence on the movement of Qi needed for digestion. Using Lv-13 is a useful way to do that whilst at the same time treating the Spleen directly.

SP-15 (Da Heng) is a local point on the abdomen that helps to move Qi throughout the intestines, and is particularly useful as a local point to relieve constipation due to blockage of the Large Intestine. Although this point is particularly good for constipation by regulating the flow of Qi within the intestines, it is also useful to treat diarrhoea due to infection or inflammation of the intestines.

SJ-6 (Zhi Gou) is a distal point that is famous for circulating Qi and fluids through the intestines. This function makes it a particularly good point for patients suffering from constipation due to Heat and Dryness within the intestines.

ST-36 (Zu San Li) is listed as one of Gao Wu's command points. It is listed specifically as the command point for the abdomen, meaning it should be used for any condition stemming from issues within the abdomen. It is also a very strong tonifying point for both the Stomach and the Spleen, helping to rectify the functions of the digestive system.

P-6 (Nei Guan) is also listed as one of the command points, added later to Gao Wu's original four. It is listed as the command point for the Heart, Chest and Epigastrium, and is excellent for treating rebellious Qi in the Stomach in addition to treating food retention and bloating by promoting the circulation of Qi within the torso (as part of its relationship with the Liver channel through the Jue Yin). It also helps to release the diaphragm, which as a result eases stagnation within the digestive system.

R-12 (Zhong Wan) is the Front Mu point of the Stomach, and is used for both deficiency and excess type conditions of the Stomach due to its harmonising function, in addition to tonifying the Spleen. It is an excellent point to stimulate for many digestive disorders, simply because it is the influential point of all Fu organs.

R-13 (Shang Wan) is an excellent point for treating excessive conditions of the Stomach, and encouraging the descending of the Stomach Qi for treatment of conditions such as nausea, vomiting, hiccup and belching.

Back Shu points of the Spleen (BL-20, Pi Shu), Stomach (BL-21, Wei Shu), Large Intestine (BL-25, Da Chang Shu) and the Small Intestine (BL-27, Xiao Chang Shu) are all useful for treating digestive disorders. Other Back Shu points should also be taken into account depending on the differential diagnosis, as all Back Shu points help to both release Heat from their corresponding organ and to transport Yang Qi from the Du channel to the corresponding organ when treating deficiency conditions.

Opening and regulating the abdomen

First of all, before any treatment or palpation can be done on the abdomen, it is necessary to 'open and regulate' the abdomen. This allows the connective tissues within the abdomen and lower torso to relax, releasing tension within the bowels and digestive organs, consequently allowing space for the Qi, Blood and Body Fluids to flow smoothly throughout. Opening and regulating the abdomen before anything else will make palpation diagnosis easier and enable any treatment performed locally or distally to have a greater effect due to the channels and pathways flowing better and more efficiently. Doing this alone can often rectify many conditions related to the abdomen. To open and regulate the abdomen:

- Begin by gently opening the Qi Men within the joints of the hips, pelvis and lower spine using the techniques **Yao Fa** and **Ba Shen Fa** (stagnation can occur within this area from both standing upright and prolonged sitting, affecting all of the channels that enter and exit the abdomen from the lower body and extremities).

- Perform **Mo Fa** and **Rou Fa** lightly on the abdomen to simply warm and activate the area, and to get the patient to feel comfortable and used to touch. This should be done in a clockwise direction whilst standing on the right of the patient (to encourage the direction of the digestive system).

- Once the abdomen begins to relax, apply a little more pressure using **Rou Fa** to begin moving the tissues beneath the surface, and apply **Tui Fa** across the abdomen slowly with the palm root. *All movements should be gentle and steady to help the patient feel relaxed.*

- After a few minutes of relaxing the tissues, it is necessary to stimulate movement within the abdomen. Do this by pressing the eight directions around the navel (approximately 3 cun from the navel in each of the eight compass directions – see the illustration below) starting with North (directly below the navel). Stimulate each of the points using **An Fa** with the fingers or thumb. *The direction of pressure should be towards the spine and each point should be pressed for only a few seconds.* As each point is pressed, **Rou Fa** can be applied in a clockwise direction to stimulate the point further. This sequence should only be done once, as it can strongly move the Qi through the intestines.

- Now that the abdominal tissues have been relaxed and movement has been created, release tension from around walls of the navel by applying pressure again in the eight directions using **An Fa** to apply pressure, again for just a few seconds. *The direction of pressure should be 45 degrees down and out from the centre into the walls of the navel.*

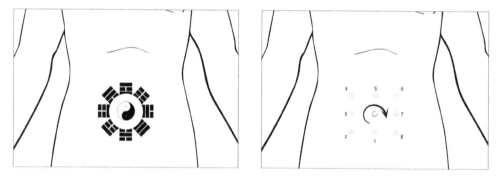

The eight abdominal directions

Abdominal palpation and release techniques

Once the abdomen has been activated using the sequence above, it will be much easier to find issues within the abdomen when using palpation. When palpating the abdomen, we are looking for Ashi points (as described in Section 2) of any kind that may indicate emotional and/or physical stagnation.

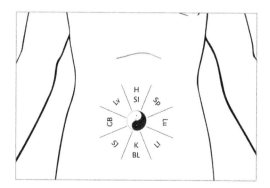

The eight abdominal zones

To palpate the abdomen, we use the tips of our fingers, and again divide the abdomen up into eight zones. We begin in the North direction (which is below the navel), and work clockwise, palpating for any areas of soreness or tension. Once we come across an area of soreness or tension, we take a mental or physical note, and move on to the next zone. We palpate all eight zones in order, taking note of any issues.

Once we have palpated each of the eight zones, we start back at the North direction and use a combination of **Rou Fa, An Fa** and **Tui Fa** to massage and release any tension that we found whilst palpating. The direction of pressure and massage should now be performed towards the navel, as this is said to be where abdominal tension can be released energetically. Once we have massaged and released all eight zones, we return to palpation again to note any changes. We apply this entire sequence of palpating and releasing a total of three times if necessary.

Constipation

Constipation is a common complaint in the West, and is characterised by infrequency in bowel movement, inability to pass stools with ease or inability to fully empty the bowels. From a Chinese Medicine perspective, the most common patterns appearing with constipation include Qi stagnation, Heat (causing dryness of the intestines) or Blood/Yin deficiency (again, causing dryness of the intestines). Each of these patterns cause lack of movement and peristalsis within the bowels, leading to constipation, and are most commonly due to dietary or emotional factors.

To treat constipation, once the sequence for opening and regulating the abdomen has been applied, perform the following sequence:

Supine position

- Use **Fen Tui Fa** at the lower boarder of the ribs to help release the diaphragm on both sides and move downward towards the level of the navel.

- Use **Rou Fa** with the palm root clockwise around the navel nine times.

- Use **Yi Zhi Chan Tui Fa** or **Rou Fa** with the thumb to stimulate SP-15 (Da Heng) and ST-25 (Tian Shu) for 1–2 minutes each.

- Again, use **Rou Fa** with the palm root clockwise around the navel nine times.

- Use **Rou Fa** with the thumb to stimulate Lv-13 (Zhang Men).

Prone position

- Warm the lower back using **Mo Fa**, then use **Gun Fa** and **Rou Fa** on the lower back, focusing on stimulating BL-21 (Wei Shu), BL-22 (San Jiao Shu) and BL-25 (Da Chang Shu).

- Use **Ca Fa** on the lower back to create warmth and expansion followed by **Pai Fa** and **Ji Fa** to dissipate any stagnation.

- Finish with **Ba Shen Fa** on the lower back and hips.

After-care advice

- In order to encourage the movement of Qi and Body Fluids throughout the abdomen and the intestines, it is important to advise the patient on good posture whilst eating, and to encourage gentle movement shortly after meals. Additionally, patients should eat when they are relaxed and take sufficient time for a meal. It is also best for the patient to wait if they are in an excessive emotional state, feel stressed, hurried or are on the go. The best way to eat is to smell the food (engage the Spleen through the Lungs), sit down (away from any project or task at hand), relax and enjoy the meal, while concentrating on chewing well.

Modifications according to syndrome differentiation

The following techniques and suggestions may be added to the above routine according to the syndrome differentiation:

Qi stagnation

- Use **Gun Fa** along the top of the shoulders and use **An Fa** perpendicularly to stimulate GB-21 (Jian Jing) to descend the Qi.

- Use **Cuo Fa** on the intercostals whilst the patient is in a seated position.

- Use **Yi Zhi Chan Tui Fa** or **Rou Fa** with the thumb to stimulate GB-34 (Yang Ling Quan), Lv-3 (Tai Chong) and LI-4 (He Gu).

Blood and/or Yin deficiency

- Use **Yi Zhi Chan Tui Fa** or **Rou Fa** with the thumb to stimulate SJ-6 (Zhi Gou) and K-6 (Zhao Hai) for 1–2 minutes each.

- Use **Cuo Fa** on the lower extremities to open the Yin channels of the legs.

- It is important to discuss dietary advice for patients with Blood or Yin deficiency.

Heat

- Use **Yi Zhi Chan Tui Fa** or **Rou Fa** with the thumb to stimulate LI-4 (He Gu) and LI-11 (Qu Chi) for 1–2 minutes each.

- Use **Gun Fa** on the Bladder channel, focusing on BL-21 (Wei Shu) down to BL-27 (Xiao Chang Shu).

Diarrhoea

Diarrhoea is characterised as having an increased frequency of bowel movements that pass loose or watery stools with or without urgency. From a Chinese Medicine perspective, diarrhoea is most commonly due to Cold and deficient type patterns, such as Spleen Qi/Yang deficiency, Spleen and Kidney Yang deficiency or a complex pattern such as Liver invading the Spleen. Diarrhoea may also be due to excess pathogens such as Damp Heat, which is most commonly due to infection or food poisoning.

To treat diarrhoea, once the sequence for opening and regulating the abdomen has been applied, perform the following sequence:

Supine position

- Use **Gun Fa** and **Rou Fa** upwards along the thigh aspect of the Stomach and Spleen Sinew channels.

- Use **Yi Zhi Chan Tui Fa** or **Rou Fa** (with the thumb) to stimulate ST-36 (Zu San Li) and SP-6 (San Yin Jiao) for 1–2 minutes each.

- Use **Ca Fa** with the fingers along the Ren channel from R-12 (Zhong Wan) to R-4 (Guan Yuan) for 2–3 minutes to warm the abdomen.

- Use **Ca Fa** with the palm horizontally across the abdomen at the level of SP-15 (Da Heng) and just below for 2–3 minutes.

- Use **Yi Zhi Chan Tui Fa** to stimulate ST-25 (Tian Shu) for 1–2 minutes.

Prone position

- Use **Mo Fa** and **Rou Fa** to warm the back, including the lower back, and to open the channels.

- Use **Gun Fa** along the Bladder channel at the lower back and sacrum, focusing on BL-20 (Pi Shu), BL-21 (Wei Shu) and BL-25 (Da Chang Shu).

- Finish with **Ca Fa** along the Du channel from DU-14 (Da Zhui) to DU-4 (Ming Men) for 2–3 minutes.

After-care advice

- Whether the diarrhoea is caused by a deficiency of Qi/Yang or by excess pathogens within the body, the Spleen needs to be nourished and looked after by not overwhelming it with activity. This means that foods that are difficult to digest, such as raw foods or foods that are cold in nature should be avoided.

Any salads should be lightly steamed. Plain cooked meals are preferred, such as the ones based on rice, carrots and lean meat, as well as broth. It is also important to eat little and often, ideally warm meals, again to avoid overwhelming the body's digestive system, and have a larger meal in the morning when the Stomach and Spleen are at their most active.

Modifications according to syndrome differentiation

The following techniques and suggestions may be added to the above routine according to the syndrome differentiation:

Spleen Qi and/or Yang deficiency

- Use **An Fa** with the palm to press firmly up the thigh aspect of the Spleen channel from SP-10 (Xue Hai) to SP-12 (Chong Men).

- Use **Yi Zhi Chan Tui Fa** or **Rou Fa** with the thumb to stimulate SP-3 (Tai Bai).

- Moxibustion is essential in order to tonify Yang.

Kidney Yang deficiency

- Use **Ca Fa** on the lower lumbar at the level of BL-23 (Shen Shu) and DU-4 (Ming Men) until enough heat is generated.

- Use **Cuo Fa** on the foot and Ca Fa on K-1 (Yong Quan) until enough heat is generated.

- Moxibustion is essential in order to tonify Yang.

Liver invading the Spleen

- Use **Cuo Fa** on the intercostals whilst the patient is in a seated position.

- Use **Yi Zhi Chan Tui Fa** or **Rou Fa** with the thumb to stimulate Lv-3 (Tai Chong) and Lv-13 (Zhang Men).

Damp Heat in the Large Intestine

- Use gentle **Pai Fa** on the lower abdomen.

- Use **Pai Fa** followed by **Ji Fa** on the lower back, focusing on BL-25 (Da Chang Shu).

- Use **Yi Zhi Chan Tui Fa** or **Rou Fa** to stimulate SP-9 (Yin Ling Quan) and LI-11 (Qu Chi).

Food retention

Classically, a Tui Na practitioner would use the emesis (vomiting) method of treatment along with Herbal Medicine to help break up food stagnations to relieve food retention. Whereas using Herbal Medicine (such as the formula Bao He Wan) is a good idea, it is best to avoid using the emesis method if possible (explained in Section 1) for obvious reasons. If the food retention is severe, we may get the patient to use the emesis method themselves by putting their fingers down their throat or drinking a salt water solution to cause the gag reflex and induce vomiting. However, if the food retention is not so severe, the following method can help to resolve it.

To treat food retention, once the sequence for opening and regulating the abdomen has been applied, perform the following sequence:

Supine position

- Use **An Fa** on R-13 (Shang Wan) with pressure applied obliquely towards R-8.
- Use **Yi Zhi Chan Tui Fa** or **Rou Fa** with the thumb to stimulate P-6 (Nei Guan).
- Use **Tui Fa** along the Ren channel from R-13 (Shang Wan) to the navel.
- Use **Mo Fa** in a clockwise direction on the epigastrium for 2–3 minutes or until warmth is felt.

Prone position

- Use **Mo Fa** and **Rou Fa** to warm the back, including the lower back, and to open the channels.
- Use **Pai Fa** followed by **Ji Fa** around the regions of BL-21 (Wei Shu).
- Use **Yao Fa** on the waist and lower lumbar.

After-care advice

- For patients with food retention, it is important that they are advised to eat slowly. Eating at a slower pace and chewing the food sufficiently will give time for the Stomach to digest better to prevent further food retention. What's more, they need to eat the last meal a few hours before bedtime. Similar to the advice given to those with constipation, it is important to advise the patient on good posture whilst eating, and to encourage gentle movement shortly after meals. This will help reduce any potential stagnation. Lastly, it is important to not engage in any mental activity during eating, as this puts extra demand on the Stomach due to the need to digest and process 'information' in addition to the food.

Chapter 14

Gynaecological Disorders

Gynaecology is a hugely broad area of medicine, from both Western and Chinese Medicine perspectives. It relies on knowledge of many specific diagnostic patterns and health conditions in addition to requiring a deeper understanding of female physiology. It is a huge topic containing many factors in its own right, with several books specialising in this topic alone. However, within Chinese Medicine, it is considered to be imperative that the menstrual cycle is regulated first and foremost in the treatment of any gynaecological disorder. This lays the foundation of any gynaecological treatment. This section therefore focuses on regulating the menstrual cycle with Tui Na, as doing so can often help a great deal with most gynaecological conditions without needing to go any further.

Key acupressure points

Although it is important to choose acupressure points according to their functions and indications in respect to your Chinese Medicine differential diagnosis, the following points are just a few that are especially regarded for their use in regulating the reproductive system:

LU-7 (Lie Que) is the master point of the Ren Mai (Conception vessel), and is therefore used to open and regulate the Ren Mai. It also helps the Kidneys to circulate Jing throughout the body, and is used to help the body to release emotion (especially grief and sense of loss, both of which are often experienced with infertility) by 'releasing the exterior'.

ST-29 (Gui Lai) helps to regulate the menses by directing Qi and Blood to the Uterus. It is also useful in Tui Na as it can be used to engage the broad ligament and help with gentle alignment of the Uterus.

SP-4 (Gong Sun) is the master point of the Chong Mai (Penetrating vessel), and is therefore used to open and activate the Chong Mai and influence Blood (as the Chong Mai is the 'Sea of Blood'). SP-4 is also used to strengthen the Spleen's function of holding the Blood, and should be used if there is heavy Blood flow due to a deficiency of the Spleen Qi.

SP-6 (San Yin Jiao) is the meeting point of the Liver, Kidney and Spleen channels. It is therefore excellent for regulating the menses due to the influences the three channels have on gynaecology. It also causes the Uterus and cervix to contract, and should therefore not be used during pregnancy or menstruation (unless in the presence of excessive bleeding).

SP-8 (Di Ji) is the Xi-Cleft point on the Spleen channel, and is used to 'regulate the menses'. It is considered to be an important point for regulating the flow of Qi and Blood within the lower Jiao by treating and preventing stagnation of Qi and Blood.

SP-10 (Xue Hai) has a regulating and cooling effect on the Blood, and is therefore used for heavy periods when there is Heat in the Blood. It also has a moving effect on the Blood, so is often used during times when the Blood is required to move such as during the menstrual period.

BL-17 (Ge Shu), BL-18 (Gan Shu) and BL-20 (Pi Shu) are known classically as the 'Six Gentlemen', and are used as a combination for Blood deficiency. Bl-17 is the influential point of Blood, whereas BL-18 and BL-20 are the Back Shu (transport) points of the Liver (which stores the Blood) and Spleen (which produces the Blood) respectively.

BL-23 (Shen Shu) is the Back Shu point of the Kidney, and is used to transport Yang Qi directly from the Du Mai to the Kidneys. It is an excellent point used to treat any chronic deficiency of the Kidneys.

BL-24 (Qi Hai Shu) is the Back Shu point of the 'Sea of Qi', and is also commonly referred to unofficially as the Uterus Shu point. It directs Yang Qi directly from the Du Mai to the lower Dan Tian, and also the region where the Uterus is located. It can be used to help regulate the Uterus and regulate the menses.

K-3 (Tai Xi), K-6 (Zhang Hai) and K-7 (Fu Liu) are all points used for tonifying and nourishing the Kidneys. K-3 is the Yuan-Source point of the Kidney channel, and can be used to tonify both the Kidney Qi and Yang in addition to nourishing the Kidney Yin and Jing. K-6, on the other hand, is considered to have a greater effect on the Kidney Yin by activating the Yin fluids of the Kidneys, whereas K-7 is considered to have a greater effect on the Kidney Yang.

K-13 (Qi Xue) and K-14 (Si Man) are points that both sit locally to the Uterus and strengthen the Kidneys. K-13 has a more nourishing and consolidating effect on the Qi and Jing, whereas K-14 has a more moving aspect on the Qi and is used to encourage the circulation of Qi and Blood within the Uterus.

R-4 (Guan Yuan) and R-6 (Qi Hai) act similarly to K-13 (Qi Xue) and K-14 (Si Man) above, in that they act to consolidate and move respectively. R-4 is used to draw in Qi and Blood to the Uterus and consolidate the Yin and Jing to nourish the Tian Gui, whereas R-6 is used to activate the Dan Tian which in turn tonifies the Qi and circulates Qi and Blood within the lower Jiao. Both are excellent points to both nourish and regulate the Uterus.

DU-3 (Yao Yang Guan) and DU-4 (Ming Men) are both located on the lumbar spine, and are used during the Yang phase of the menstrual cycle or when there is Cold in the Uterus. DU-3 directs Yang Qi directly to the Uterus and 'warms the Chamber of Blood', which is a classical name given to the Uterus. DU-4, on the other hand, activates the Ming Men Fire, and is used to invigorate the Yang of the whole body.

EX-M-CA-18 (Zi Gong) is an empirical point located 3 cun lateral and 4 cun below the navel. Its name can be translated as 'Child Palace', and it is related to the effect the point has on the ovaries. Zi Gong is an excellent point to stimulate the ovaries, regulate Qi and Blood within the Uterus, and help to align the Uterus by activating the round ligaments.

The four phases of the menstrual cycle

In order to help better understand the female physiology and reproductive process, the menstrual cycle was classically split into two key phases according to Yin and Yang – the Yin phase (menstruation to ovulation) and the Yang phase (ovulation to menstruation). The Yin phase is characterised by substance and form. It is governed by Blood, nourishment of the follicles and uterine lining, and the filling of the Ren and Chong Mai. It is during this stage of the cycle that the foundations are laid and put in place ready for ovulation and fertilisation to take place. The Yang phase, on the other hand, is characterised by warmth, movement and generation. The Yang phase is governed by Qi and is responsible for providing a suitable environment for the fertilised egg to implant in addition to promoting life – if pregnancy does indeed occur, it is the Yang that is responsible for the rapid growth and development of the embryo during this time.

'Without Yang, Yin cannot transform; without Yin, Yang cannot generate' – the basic theories of Yin and Yang tell us that in order for the Yin phase to transform into the Yang phase, there needs to be a sufficient build-up of Yin, and vice versa. This is an important concept to understand in regards to the menstrual cycle (and Chinese Medicine as a whole). If there is a problem with one part of the cycle, it is essential to look at and treat other aspects of a cycle in order to build a strong foundation. For example, should the Yin be deficient and not grow sufficiently during the Yin phase, then there will be a weak foundation on which the Yang phase can build. This may cause issues in the onset of the Yang phase, thus causing delayed ovulation. A similar concept within Chinese Medicine would be to treat Winter diseases in the Summer (*Dong Bing Xia Zhi*, 冬病夏治).

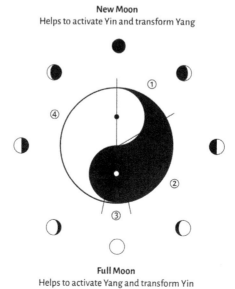

New Moon
Helps to activate Yin and transform Yang

Full Moon
Helps to activate Yang and transform Yin

The four phases of the menstrual cycle

The four phases of the menstrual cycle and the movements of Yin and Yang

Phase One: Menstruation – Extreme Yang transforms into Yin.

Phase Two: Post-period (follicular) – Yin waxes whilst Yang wanes.

Phase Three: Ovulation – Extreme Yin transforms into Yang.

Phase Four: Pre-period (luteal) – Yang waxes whilst Yin wanes.

As Chinese Medicine developed and understanding of internal medicine grew, the phases of the menstrual cycle were advanced into *four* key phases. The four phase theory has since been taken further in modern Chinese Medicine by famous physician Dr Xia Gucheng. He pioneered the use of the four phases of the menstrual cycle to understand the female cycle based on the movements of Qi and Blood and the actions of Yin and Yang. The four phases can also be used to help guide treatment principles and offer lifestyle advice. These four phases are menstruation (Yang transforming to Yin), the follicular/post-menstrual phase (Yin waxing), ovulation (Yin transforming to Yang) and the luteal phase (Yang waxing). In the treatment of female infertility, and gynaecological conditions in general, it is essential to understand the mechanisms of each of the four phases in order to understand what issues may possibly be affecting menstrual health and also to know what substances need treating at the specific times. It must be noted, however, that treatment according to the four phases of the menstrual cycle should only be used as a foundation to the treatment, and treatment according to any overlying or underlying factors must still be given according to individual syndrome differentiation.

Correcting structural issues of the uterus

Tui Na can indeed be used to fix structural issues of the uterus and ovaries, such as a retro-verted uterus and ovary misalignment. These manipulation techniques are a little more complex and cannot simply be explained in a book, and should be observed in practice due to the nature of applied pressure. The following procedures should be used to help regulate the cycle in cases of non-structural gynecological conditions; however, they may also be used to help mild structural issues.

Phase One: Menstruation

Phase one of the menstrual cycle is known classically as extreme Yang transforming into Yin, also known as 'double Yang transforming to Yin'. This is the part of the cycle where the Yin is activated and the body 'gets rid of the old to start with the new'. In Western terms, this stage of the cycle is known as 'menstruation' or the 'menstrual period'. Phase One is said to take place during days 1–5 based on a standard 28-day cycle, and was classically divided into a further five phases based on the promotion (Sheng) cycle of the Five Phases (Wu Xing), starting with the Water element (discussed further below regarding emotional release through menstruation).

It is during Phase One that the Ren and Chong Mai begin to empty due to the downward pull of the Yin energy, allowing the menstrual Blood (Tian Gui Shui, 天癸水) to flow downwards and to exit the body. During this process, the uterine lining (endometrium) is shed due to lack of fertilisation, and expelled from the Uterus via the cervix and the vagina. This phase is also considered to be the 'Blood' phase of the cycle due to the focus on regulating the movement and mechanisms of Blood during this time. Due to Phase One being dominated by Blood and the loss of Blood, there may be an increase in dreaming and also fatigue or sleepiness during this time and shortly after, as the Hun may not be anchored correctly within the Blood. Therefore, women should rest and find peaceful activities whilst keeping exercise and exertion to a minimum until the Blood has been replenished during the next phase.

Treatment principles during this phase are to encourage the movement of Blood and to regulate Qi in order for a smooth flow and release of menstrual Blood. Should the menses be scanty, it is important to strongly move Blood to ensure that a full release occurs so that there is no 'old' or stagnant blood present during the following cycle. When Blood is not moving sufficiently, there may be signs of discomfort and/or menstrual cramping. Should there be an excessive amount of Blood flow, however, or if the duration of bleeding is too long, treatment should be aimed towards slowing down the flow and/or stopping bleeding. Treatment during this phase is often aimed towards the Liver and Spleen due to their actions on the Qi and Blood, and activating the Chong Mai.

The release of emotion

Phase One of the menstrual cycle additionally has an increased importance, as it is closely linked to the letting go of emotions through the Blood during menstruation. It is significant in regards to the emotional release of a woman. It is through the connection between the Heart and Uterus via the Bao Mai that enables the female to release what could be considered as 'emotional debris' through the monthly release of menstrual Blood. As emotions are considered to exist within the Blood from a Chinese Medicine perspective, it is important for the connection between the Heart and the Uterus to be fully open, and for the female to bleed for long enough and smoothly enough to enable a full release of emotional pathogens. This helps to get rid of any residual emotions that may have built up over the previous month, or longer. Treatment of the Heart and Pericardium is therefore also important during this phase of the menstrual cycle to allow a release of emotions and opening up the Bao Mai in addition to the treatment principles discussed above.

If period signs arise at certain times during the cycle, such as heavier bleeding or cramping, it may indicate an issue with a particular part of the emotional release. The five (or so) days of the period can be split into five energetic stages, and the emotions that are released during these times are as follows:

Stage One: Water/Zhi – Fears and insecurities

Stage Two: Wood/Hun – Anger, resentment and frustration

Stage Three: Fire/Shen – Mania and excitation

Stage Four: Earth/Yi – Worries and obsessive thoughts

Stage Five: Metal/Po – Grief, sadness and attachments

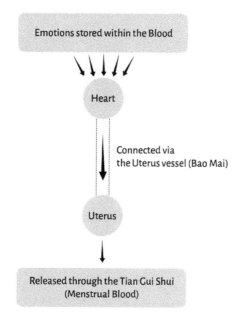

Emotional release from the Heart via the Menstrual Blood

Tui Na prescription for Phase One of the menstrual cycle (Menstruation)

- With the patient lying in prone, begin by opening and activating the Chong Mai by stimulating SP-4 (Gong Sun) on the right and P-6 (Nei Guan) on the left with **Yi Zhi Chan Tui Fa** for 1–2 minutes each. Once the Chong Mai has been activated, use **Gun Fa** and **Rou Fa** for 4–5 minutes on the lower back and sacrum to stimulate the Uterus and move Qi and Blood in the lower Jiao. Focus on stimulating specific points such as BL-23 (Shen Shu), BL-24 (Qi Hai Shu) and DU-3 (Yao Yang Guan). Finish by using gentle **Pai Fa** on the lower back to encourage dissipation of any stasis or stagnation.

- With the patient lying in a supine position, gently open the Qi Men within the joints of the hips and pelvis by using **Yao Fa** and **Ba Shen Fa** (stagnation can occur within this area from both standing upright and prolonged sitting, affecting downward flow of menstrual Blood).

- Use a combination of **An Fa**, **Gun Fa** and **Rou Fa** along the leg aspects of the Spleen and Liver Sinew channels, followed by using **Cuo Fa** down each leg to help open the Yin channels.

- Use **An Fa** or **Rou Fa** to stimulate SP-10 (Xue Hai) and Lv-3 (Tai Chong) for 1–2 minutes each to encourage the movement of Blood. *If the bleeding is excessive* (too heavy or prolonged), use **An Fa** or **Rou Fa** to stimulate SP-6 (San Yin Jiao). *If the period is painful,* use **An Fa** or **Rou Fa** to stimulate SP-8 (Di Ji).

- Gently warm the lower abdomen with **Mo Fa** and Ca Fa for 2–3 minutes to encourage movement of Qi and Blood, followed by using Ca Fa with the fingers up and down the Ren channel from R-14 (Ju Que) to the navel 108 times. Use **An Fa** or **Rou Fa** to stimulate ST-29 (Gui Lai) to assist the movement of Blood within the lower Jiao and Uterus.

- Use **Rou Fa** in a wave-type motion on the whole abdomen to encourage the free flow of Qi between the middle and lower Jiao. Stimulate R-14 (Ju Que) with **Yi Zhi Chan Tui Fa** for 1–2 minutes, followed by stimulating R-12 (Zhong Wan) with **Rou Fa** in a downward direction for 1–2 minutes.

- Ask the patient to take a deep breath, and use **An Fa** (or **Ya Fa**) with the fingers or hypothenar eminence on R-4 (Guan Yuan) to deeply suppress as the patient breathes out. Hold the position for 1–2 seconds, then release quickly to mobilise and quicken the flow Qi and Blood. Repeat this three times followed by **Ca Fa** to disperse any stagnation.

- To open the connection between the Heart and Uterus (for a smooth release of emotional debris through the menstrual Blood), warm the Ren Mai with **Ca Fa** from R-17 (Shan Zhong) to R-4 (Guan Yuan).

- To finish, use **An Fa** to stimulate P-6 (Nei Guan) bi-laterally to open up the chest and descend Qi and Blood through to the lower Jiao, followed by gently holding K-1 (Yong Quan) for 1–2 minutes to further encourage the downward movement of the menstrual Blood.

- Cupping on the lower abdomen and/or lower back may be used if there are Blood stasis signs, such as dark Blood with clots and pain or cramping.

Treatment principles

- Regulate Qi and Blood and move Blood (stop bleeding if it is excessive).

- Treatment is aimed primarily at regulating the Liver, Spleen and opening the Chong Mai.

- Treatment of the Heart and Pericardium is important to connect the Heart and Uterus and allow the release of emotional debris through the menstrual Blood.

After-care advice

- Increase rest and get gentle exercise (such as walking and stretching).

- Mentally 'switch off' – reduce mental activity and avoid excessive emotions to help keep the Heart and Bao Mai open.

- Avoid too much meat as this can cause stagnation; eat broths and stews to aid the Spleen's digestion, and eat little and often to avoid stagnation.

Phase Two: The Follicular Phase

Phase Two of the menstrual cycle is known classically as the Yin waxing phase. This is the Yin part of the cycle where Yin grows and develops between the end of menstruation and the beginning of ovulation, and is said to take place during days 6–13 based on a standard 28-day cycle. In Western terms, this may be noted as the 'post-menstrual' or 'follicular phase'.

During Phase Two, the Blood and Yin are initially deficient due to the loss of menstrual blood (Tian Gui Shui) during the five or so days of menstruation, and the Ren and Chong Mai have been relatively emptied. The body during this time is working on replenishing the Blood that has been lost through menstruation, and also nourishing the Yin whilst the Ren and Chong Mai refill ready for the third phase (ovulation). The Kidney Yin directs nourishment towards the Uterus and the uterine lining begins to develop again and cervical fluid begins to increase. This phase is considered to be the Yin phase of the cycle, and it is important during this phase to ensure that Yin has been nourished enough to provide a strong enough foundation on which Yang can build from. Yin is considered to be the fuel to the fire of Yang. If there is not enough fuel, then the fire will not be strong enough and may fail to activate ovulation (when Yin transforms to Yang). It is this stage of the cycle that is often the reason that a woman's menstrual cycle varies in length. For example, if this phase goes beyond day 14, which is the time when ovulation should generally occur, then it could indicate that the body's Yin is struggling to develop sufficiently and unable to transform to Yang in time.

Treatment principles for Phase Two should be focused on nourishing Yin and regulating Blood, in addition to supporting the Ren and Chong Mai. Towards the end of Phase Two, Yang should also be supported in order to encourage the activation and transformation of Yin into Yang. Treatment during this phase is often aimed towards the Kidneys and Liver in order to nourish the Yin and Blood respectively. Treatment of the Stomach and Spleen may also be necessary as the foundation to post-natal Qi and to encourage the production of Blood and help to support the Kidneys through their post-natal/pre-natal relationship.

Tui Na prescription for Phase Two of the menstrual cycle (Follicular Phase)

Treatment during this phase should be much more gentle to encourage nourishment of the Yin:

- With the patient lying in a relaxed supine position, gently open the Qi Men within the joints of the hips and pelvis by using **Yao Fa** and **Ba Shen Fa**. This will help the effectiveness of distal point stimulation.

- Open and activate the Ren Mai by stimulating LU-7 (Lie Que) on the right and K-6 (Zhao Hai) on the left with **Yi Zhi Chan Tui Fa** or **Rou Fa** for 1–2 minutes each. Once the Ren Mai has been activated, use Ca Fa with the fingers up and down the abdomen along the Ren Mai, followed by **Yi Zhi Chan Tui Fa** on R-4 (Guan Yuan) to gather Qi and Blood towards the Uterus and to nourish the Yin Qi.

- Use a combination of **An Fa**, **Rou Fa** and **Gun Fa** on the leg aspects of the Liver, Spleen and Kidney Sinew channels. This is to help nourish the Uterus with Yin Qi in addition to regulating the Blood. Stimulate SP-6 (San Yin Jiao) using **Rou Fa** with the thumb for 1–2 minutes to help further activate the Liver, Kidney and Spleen channels.

- Ask the patient to turn on to their front and lie in a relaxed prone position. Use a combination of **Gun Fa** and **Rou Fa** on the back to open the Bladder Sinew channel, and use **An Fa** or **Rou Fa** with the thumbs to stimulate the 'Six Gentlemen' (BL-17 Ge Shu, BL-18 Gan Shu and BL-20 Pi Shu) to nourish the Blood.

- To finish, use **Tui Fa** with the 'Tiger's Mouth' to dredge down the whole body, ending with **Na Fa** to grasp K-3 (Tai Xi) and BL-60 (Kun Lun) behind the ankles. This helps to draw down and root the Qi. Repeat this six times on each side.

- *If the patient is coming up to Phase Three*, use **Ca Fa** over the Spine to activate the Du channel and assist in the transformation of Yin to Yang. Finish off by using **Mo Fa** to warm the lower back, focusing on DU-4 (Ming Men) for 2–3 minutes.

Treatment principles

- Nourish Yin and regulate Blood to replenish the Ren and Chong Mai.

- Support Yang towards the end of the phase to help the transformation from Yin to Yang.

- Treatment is aimed primarily at the Liver and Kidneys.

- The Stomach and Spleen should be strengthened to aid in the production of Blood.

After-care advice

- Begin to increase the amount of exercise.

- Eat Yin and Blood-nourishing foods – dark greens and algae are good during this phase due to their Yin and Jing supporting properties. Eat eggs, nuts and seeds, and begin to introduce more meat such as beef in order to build Blood. Also eat bland grains such as quinoa to support the Spleen.

Phase Three: Ovulation

Phase Three of the menstrual cycle is known classically as extreme Yin transforming into Yang, also known as 'double Yin transforming to Yang'. This is the part of the cycle where the Yin is full enough to provide a suitable foundation for Yang to develop upon and the Ren and Chong Mai are full enough in order to activate Tian Gui (天癸) and therefore ovulation and enable conception if necessary. In Western terms, this stage of the cycle is known as 'ovulation' or the 'mid-cycle phase' and is the shortest of the four phases lasting only a couple of days, from days 11–15 based on a standard 28-day cycle. It is during this time that the body temperature will rise slightly in accordance to the activation of Yang, and there will be a surge in the hormones LH (luteinizing hormone) and FSH (follicle stimulating hormone) that triggers the release of an egg from the ovaries. As the Yin is at its extreme, oestrogen levels peak within the body, the cervical fluids have become thicker and turned to cervical mucous, and the uterine lining is becoming thick enough for implantation of a fertilised egg.

In order to promote the transformation of Yin to Yang, it is important to nourish the Jing during this time. Jing is the fuel to the Ming Men Fire as Yin is the fuel to the Yang. The Ming Men Fire is needed for the release of the egg during menstruation, and then to warm the Uterus to provide a suitable environment for fertilisation and implantation. Phase Three is the time where Yang begins to rise, so it is important to stimulate growth of Yang. During this short phase it is vitally important to avoid raw foods or over-consumption of cold foods and liquids (cold in property or physical temperature). This is because they can be difficult for the Spleen to digest alone and would require Yang Qi to be drawn from the Kidneys to assist in the digestion of the foods.

Treatment principles during Phase Three should be aimed towards supporting and warming the Kidneys in order to nourish the Jing and to activate Yang. Treatment should also include activating and regulating the Du Mai, as the 'Sea of Yang'. This encourages the stimulation and tonification of Yang in the body. Focus on the Heart, in particular, the Heart Yang, is also essential during this time in order to open the connection between the Heart (mind) and the Uterus. This assists in the transformation from Yin to Yang, and also in the opening of the cervix and successful fertilisation of the egg as it is important to have an unrestricted flow of emotion during conception. The Shen needs to be settled and able to flow freely for there to be a good chance of successful conception.

Tui Na prescription for Phase Three of the menstrual cycle (Ovulation)

- Ask the patient to lie in a relaxed position in prone, and begin by opening and activating the Ren Mai by stimulating LU-7 (Lie Que) on the right and K-6 (Zhao Hai) on the left with **Yi Zhi Chan Tui Fa** for 1–2 minutes each. This helps to direct the Jing to the Uterus and activate ovulation.

- Generate warmth by using **Ca Fa** up and down the Du Mai, followed by using **Ca Fa** across the lower back at the level with DU-4 (Ming Men) and BL-23 (Shen Shu) to help activate Yang. Use **An Fa** to stimulate BL-24 (Qi Hai) and **Yi Zhi Chan Tui Fa** to stimulate DU-3 (Yao Yang Guan). These points transport Yang Qi directly from the Du channel to the Uterus.

- Ask the patient to turn over and lie in a relaxed supine position, and use **Mo Fa** on the lower abdomen to warm and relax the area. Place each thumb on both sides of the abdomen at the location of EX-M-CA-18 (Zi Gong) and firmly, yet comfortably, stimulate using **Rou Fa** for 1–2 minutes. This helps to bring Qi and Blood to the region to stimulate the ovaries. If there is tightness in the lower abdominal muscles, ask the patient to lift the knees up slightly to release some tension, and place a pillow or a leg bolster beneath the knees.

- Place your fingers at ST-29 (Gui Lai), pointing in the direction of R-4 (Guan Yuan). Use **An Fa** with the fingers to push into ST-29 (Gui Lai), with the pressure directed inwards and towards the top of Uterus. This should be done as the patient breathes out, holds for 2–3 seconds, then releases quickly and is repeated three times. This helps to relax and align the broad ligament that holds the Uterus in place in a neutral position.

- Use **Mo Fa** to create warmth and relaxation in the lower abdomen, followed by **Rou Fa** with both hands (one in front of the other) in a wave-like movement for 1–2 minutes.

- Finish off by warming the Ren Mai with **Ca Fa** from R-17 (Shan Zhong) to R-4 (Guan Yuan). This helps to open and stimulate the connection between the Heart and Uterus to allow a sufficient opening of the cervix ready for conception.

Treatment principles

- Nourish Jing, support Yang, open the Ren Mai and activate the Du Mai.

- Treatment should be aimed at the Kidneys in order to nourish Jing and to stimulate Yang through the Ming Men.

- A focus on the Heart is important for opening of the cervix and for conception.

After-care advice

- Begin to eat lighter foods, and avoid raw foods or salads as this damages Yang and causes contraction within the abdomen due to Cold.

- Let go of obsessive thoughts or emotions to help prevent stagnation in the next phase.

Phase Four: The Luteal Phase

Phase Four of the menstrual cycle is known classically as the Yang waxing phase. This is now the Yang part of the cycle, and it is where Yang grows and develops between ovulation and the beginning of the menstrual period. It is the longest of the four phases and takes place during days 16–28 based on a standard 28-day cycle. In Western terms, this is known as the 'luteal phase' or the 'pre-menstrual phase'. This phase does not vary in length by more than a day or two. For example, if a woman's menstrual cycle is irregular and varies in length from month to month, then it is most likely to be the Yin phase (follicular phase) that is changing in length rather than the Yang phase (luteal phase).

During Phase Four, the uterine lining continues to develop and 'ripen' for a short period under the influence of the Kidney Yang and the foundation of the Kidney Yin. Phase Four is largely dominated by Yang, and also largely governed by the free flow of Qi by the Liver. It is important for the Yang energy of the body to keep the Uterus warm and provide a suitable environment for the egg to implant and develop if fertilisation takes place. It is also this warmth that assists in drying up the cervical fluids. Should there be a deficiency of Yang, this may give rise to what is known classically as a 'Cold Uterus', which is a major cause of female infertility. It is equally essential for the Qi to flow smoothly to ensure that there is no obstruction within the Bao Mai and Bao Luo. Should there be any stagnation of the Liver Qi, then there may be discomfort leading up to or during the menstrual period. This is due to stagnation at the physical level, or pre-menstrual tension (PMT), giving rise to frustration and irritability due to constraint of the Hun on a spiritual level. Equally important, if there is stagnation of Qi prior to the menstrual period, there may be clots and cramping during menstruation due to stasis of Blood in the Uterus.

Treatment principles during Phase Four should be aimed toward supporting the Kidney Yang, warming the 'chamber of Blood' (the Uterus), and stimulating the Ming Men Fire. Warming techniques on the abdomen or the lower back, such as moxibustion or Heat lamp therapy, are often used during this phase to assist in the warming function of the Kidney Yang. Treatment should also be aimed towards relieving the Liver of any constraint and ensuring that the Qi is flowing freely throughout the body and especially within the lower Jiao.

Tui Na prescription for Phase Four of the menstrual cycle (Luteal Phase)

Treatment during this phase can be much more Yang and should be more moving to avoid any stagnation. However, if there is any chance of pregnancy, Tui Na should again be gentler and more nourishing:

- With the patient lying in a relaxed prone position, begin by opening and activating the Chong Mai by stimulating SP-4 (Gong Sun) on the right and P-6 (Nei Guan) on the left with **Yi Zhi Chan Tui Fa** for 1–2 minutes each. This is done to help prepare the Blood ready for menstruation during the next phase.

- Use **Mo Fa** and **Rou Fa** to relax and warm the lower back, followed by **Ca Fa** across the lumbar and sacral regions, focusing on DU-4 (Ming Men) and BL-23 (Shen Shu). Use **Gun Fa** and **Rou Fa** on the leg aspects of the Bladder channel to release the lower back.

- Ask the patient to take a seated position, and perform **Cuo Fa** on the intercostals for 1–2 minutes to activate the Liver and Gall Bladder. This helps to regulate the flow of Liver Qi and resolve stagnation.

- Ask the patient to lie on their back in a supine position and gently open the Qi Men within the joints of the hips and pelvis by using **Yao Fa** and **Ba Shen Fa**. Use a combination of **An Fa**, **Gun Fa** and **Rou Fa** to work up the Liver and Spleen Sinew channels.

- Use **Rou Fa** with the thumb to stimulate K-7 (Fu Liu), Lv-3 (Tai Chong) and SP-8 (Di Ji) for 1–2 minutes each.

- Use **Mo Fa** and **Rou Fa** to gently warm and relax the abdomen for 1–2 minutes. Use **Rou Fa** with the thumb and fingers to stimulate ST-29 (Gui Lai) bi-laterally at the same time (using the thumb on one side and two fingers on the other). Now use **Na Fa** to 'grasp the Uterus' in this position and gently move it from left to right. This helps to remove any stagnations and bindings of the round ligaments and broad ligament, both of which maintain the structure of the Uterus.

- Ask the patient to take a deep breath, and use **An Fa** or **Rou Fa** to deeply stimulate R-3 (Yao Yang Guan) as the patient breathes out. Hold the pressure for 4–5 seconds and release quickly to help resolve any stagnation. Repeat this three times. **Note:** This can feel uncomfortable to the patient if their bladder is full.

Treatment principles

- Tonify Yang, move Qi and regulate Liver to prevent stagnation.

- Use of warming techniques such as moxibustion and/or Heat lamp therapy is essential.

- Treatment primarily involves the Liver and Kidneys, and opening the Chong Mai to prevent Blood stasis for next phase.

After-care advice

- Keep stretching to open the joints and to regulate the Liver.

- Eat warming foods, cooked vegetables and grains.

- Eat without excessive emotion, take time to eat and eat with good posture, all to avoid stagnation.

Chapter 15

Musculoskeletal Disorders

The key to successful treatment of musculoskeletal disorders is really diagnosis, and having the ability to identify the problematic areas and channels. Pain is rarely indicative of the location of the dysfunction. No matter how good we are at the Tui Na hand techniques, we are useless if we are unable to understand the problem, and what solution we need in order to rectify the problem.

The unique advantage of Chinese Medicine (and Tui Na) compared to many conventional Western medical models is that we don't simply focus on an area of dysfunction, but look laterally across the whole body for both diagnosis and treatment. For instance, when treating plantar fasciitis, we would not focus on the sole of the foot, heel or even the calf, but we would assess and treat all the way up to the glutes and even the lower back and hips, based on channel theory. Some schools of Chinese Medicine may also treat the palm and wrist as a mirror to the foot to further increase healing. These principles give us a great healing advantage, and can often give far better results than simply focusing on such small areas. The hips are the gateways to the knees, which are also the gateways to the ankles and feet. These gateways must be open for proper healing to occur: how can I expect Qi and Blood to flow in and out of the feet if the joints at the knees and hips are compressed and blocked? Similarly, the feet are the foundations to the knees and the hips, and must be functioning and moving properly to support the knees and hips. The same principles should be taken for the shoulders, elbows and wrists. When treating the hand, for instance, in cases such as carpal tunnel syndrome, it is essential to treat the whole arm and even into the neck. We need to keep these principles in mind when treating any musculoskeletal condition, and always be mindful of Sinew channel theory.

Tissue bindings

The joints surrounding the Qi Men are also areas where the Sinew channels are likely to 'bind', and where there is more likely to be inflammation and tension within the connective tissues. Within some older traditions of Tui Na, most emphasis was put on to the binding sites of the Sinew channels, and treatment would focus on unlocking and mobilising the joints almost exclusively.

There are too many specific musculoskeletal conditions to list in this book, with many of them having very similar mechanisms for treatment. Below are a few examples of generic treatments for areas across the body that can be used as a 'base prescription' for common conditions seen in the clinic. Remember that treatment should *always* be spontaneous and adaptable.

Swelling

If there is swelling, it is best to avoid the immediate area and rather treat the immediate surrounding areas – channel theory is important here. Using Tui Na at the site of swelling can often be uncomfortable and also counterproductive, as it can drive the swelling deeper into the joints and affect the surrounding channels. Instead, it is both important and useful to use techniques such as **Tui Fa** from the edge of the swollen area along the channel in a direction away from the swelling, both towards the body and towards the extremity. This helps to open the channels and allow the swelling to dissipate and disperse naturally. It is also important that any distal or proximal joint is fully mobilised and open to allow the flow of Qi, Blood and Body Fluids to flow in and out of the area.

General headaches

When treating headaches, it is important to understand if the headache is due to an excess or a deficiency, as this will determine the order and arrangement of treatment. In simple terms, if it is an excess type headache then we want to draw Qi and Blood away from the head and use reducing methods (see Section 1). If it is a deficiency type headache, however, we want to draw Qi and Blood towards the head in addition to using tonifying methods. The overall treatment will be similar in regards to techniques used, although how they are used will change.

We also want to identify which channels are being affected and causing the headache. We can do this by asking the patient whereabouts on the head they feel discomfort (see below), and also check using channel palpation.

Headache location	Channel indications
Occipital region	Tai Yang channels
Temple region	Shao Yang channels
Frontal region	Yang Ming channels
Vertex region	Jue Yin channels (or deficiency type)
Forehead	Gall Bladder channel
Inner canthus	Bladder channel
Sinuses	Stomach or Small Intestine channel

Perform the following sequence to treat general headaches, using tonifying or reducing methods according to the type of headache.

Seated position

- Begin with **Mo Fa** on the shoulders and upper back to help warm and relax the channels entering the head, followed by using **Nian Fa** to stimulate each of the Yang channel Jing Well points – all Sinew channels that rise to the head are Yang Sinew channels. It is important that all of these channels are open and relaxed.

- Use **Gun Fa** on the top of the shoulders towards and into the neck. Place one hand on top of the head and move the head in different directions whilst using **Gun Fa** into the neck to help manipulate the tissues in different positions. This helps to shorten, lengthen and rotate the individual muscles and tendons.

- Use **Fen Tui Fa** on the upper back, followed by **Na Fa** on the trapezius muscles and the nape of the neck. When grasping the trapezius muscles, grasp the muscles away from their original position and shake (**Dou Fa**) before releasing quickly. Repeat this six times.

- Use **Ba Shen Fa** to lift the head gently and reduce any compression at the base of the skull, followed by **Yao Fa** to help mobilise the neck and head to allow for better Qi and Blood circulation in and out of the head.

Prone position

- Begin with using **Mo Fa** on the upper back and shoulders to relax and open the Sinew channels. Use **Gun Fa** and **Rou Fa** to go deeper and relax the tissues further.

- Use **Tui Fa** on the shoulders and neck, followed by **Na Fa** on the nape of the neck. Swap between using **Tui Fa** and **Na Fa** on the nape of the neck for 4–5 minutes.

- Strongly stimulate GB-20 (Feng Chi) and DU-16 (Feng Fu) with **An Fa** or **Rou Fa** with the thumb, followed by **Tui Fa** across the Bladder channel on the neck.

- Use **An Fa** down the spine at each of the Hua Tuo Jia Ji points, stimulating each point for 1–2 seconds with the patient's out breath, followed by **Fen Tui Fa** across the whole back to reduce any stagnation.

- Use **Pai Fa** followed by **Ji Fa** on the upper back to further increase the circulation of Qi and Blood.

Supine position

- Ask the patient to turn over and lie face up in a relaxed supine position. Use gentle **Ba Shen Fa** on the head and neck.

- Use **Ma Fa** from EX-M-HN-3 (Yin Tang) to DU-24 (Shen Ting), followed by EX-M-HN-3 (Yin Tang) to ST-8 (Tou Wei), and finishing with an arc from

EX-M-HN-3 (Yin Tang) to EX-M-HN-9 (Tai Yang) whilst passing through GB-14 (Yang Bai). Repeat each one nine times.

- If the patient is suffering from deficiency type headaches, finish off by using **Yi Zhi Chan Tui Fa** to stimulate DU-20 (Bai Hui) to draw Qi and Blood upwards, towards the head. If the patient is suffering from excess type headaches, finish off by using **An Fa** on GB-21 (Jian Jing) followed by K-1 (Yong Quan).

Modifications according to headache type

The following techniques and suggestions may be added to the above routine according to the headache type.

Tai Yang type

- With the patient lying on their front, use **Na Fa** on the nape of the neck, followed by **An Fa** at BL-10 (Tian Zhu), BL-11 (Da Zhu) and BL-12 (Feng Men).

Yang Ming type

- Use **Yi Zhi Chan Tui Fa** to stimulate ST-25 (Tian Shu), and **Na Fa** between the thumb and first finger to stimulate LI-4 (He Gu).
- Use **Da Yu Ji Rou Fa** on the corners of the hairline, in the region of ST-8 (Tou Wei) for 1–2 minutes.

Shao Yang type

- Use **Da Yu Ji Rou Fa** on the sides of the head and temples for 1–2 minutes.
- Use **Rou Fa** with the thumb to stimulate GB-8 (Shuai Gu), GB-43 (Xia Xi) and SJ-5 (Wai Guan).

Jue Yin type

- Use **Da Yu Ji Rou Fa** on the vertex of the head, followed by **Yi Zhi Chan Tui Fa** to stimulate DU-20 (Bai Hui), P-7 (Da Ling) and Lv-3 (Tai Chong).

General neck pain

Neck complaints are one of the most common musculoskeletal conditions seen in the Tui Na clinic. Conditions such as cervical spondylosis (arthritis of the cervical spine), stress, trauma and even the common cold or the flu all affect the neck. When treating neck pain, it is important to first rule out any red flags, such as neck fracture. Specific diagnostic tests of the neck can be found in Section 2 of this book under 'Special examinations' (Chapter 7), with a brief discussion on red flags. It is also important to assess the patient's posture – many neck complaints are due to poor posture and misdirected pressure put through the cervico-thoracic (CT) joint (C7 and T1). Ensuring that this joint is mobilised properly, and the surrounding tissues are aligned and working effectively, is vital for the treatment of any neck complaint.

The cervico-thoracic (CT) joint

The CT joint is often a cause of neck discomfort and dysfunction in neck mobility. Ensuring that this joint is mobilised properly, and the surrounding tissues are aligned and working effectively, is vital for the treatment of any neck complaint

Seated position

- Begin with using **Mo Fa** on the patient's upper back and shoulders, followed by **Gun Fa** to the top of the shoulders and into the patient's neck. Hold the head with one hand whilst performing **Gun Fa**, and move the head at different angles to get into the various layers of the neck Sinew channels.

- Whilst taking hold of the patient's forehead/vertex with one hand, use **Na Fa** and **Rou Fa** on the nape of the neck whilst again moving the head through various comfortable positions.

- Use **An Fa** to press into each of the cervical transverse processes comfortably, whilst tilting the head in the opposite direction to the force applied.

- Use **Fen Tui Fa** across the upper back, followed by **An Fa** to stimulate the Hua Tou Jia Ji points of each vertebra from T1 to T12.

- Once the neck tissues are relaxed, use **Ban Fa** on the neck to help mobilise the spine, followed by **Ba Shen Fa** and **Yao Fa** on the neck.

Prone position

- Ask the patient to lie face down in a relaxed prone position, and begin warming the shoulders, upper back and mid back with **Mo Fa** and **Gun Fa**. Stimulate the Hua Tuo Jia Ji points with **An Fa** from T1 to T12.

- Swap between using **Rou Fa** and **Gun Fa** to relax the tissues for 5–10 minutes, working deeper as the tissues adapt. Move around the patient to access different areas at different angles.

- If there is restricted movement caused by lack of mobility within the thoracic spine, use **An Ya Fu Wei Fa**. Ensure that you work with the patient's breath. Use **Mo Fa** and **Rou Fa** to help relax any tension caused by the movement of any joints.

- Use **Tui Fa** across the Bladder and Gall Bladder Sinew channels on the neck for 3–5 minutes, followed by using **Tui Fa** down the Bladder and Du channel from the base of the occiput to the level of the junction of C7 and T1.

- Use **Na Fa** combined with **Rou Fa** on the nape of the neck and the top of the shoulders, followed by using **An Fa** to stimulate GB-20 (Feng Chi) and DU-16 (Feng Fu).

- Use **Rou Fa** and **Gun Fa** to again work on the upper and mid back for 4–5 minutes, followed by **Pai Fa** and **Ji Fa** to improve the circulation of Qi and Blood.

Supine position

- Use **Tui Fa** down the sternocleidomastoid six times, followed by **An Fa** on GB-21 (Jian Jing) for 3–5 seconds as the patient breathes out, then **Tui Fa** again down the sternocleidomastoid, this time with the patient's head to one side. Repeat this on both sides.

- Use **Ba Shen Fa** on the patient's neck, followed by moving the head to one side and pushing down on the opposite shoulder. Repeat this on each side three times, followed by lifting the patient's head forward with their neck in a comfortable flexed position. Hold this position for a few seconds.

- Finish with **Nian Fa** and **Ba Shen Fa** on each finger to stimulate the Jing Well points and help to relax each channel, followed by **Dou Fa**. Repeat this on each arm.

General lower back pain

When treating lower back pain, it is important to look at the Sinew channel pathways, and assess whether it is the Bladder, Stomach or Gall Bladder Sinew channels that are dysfunctional. Although it is important to work on all three lower Yang channels when treating general lower back pain, it is necessary to asses which channel(s) is dysfunctional so that more focus can be placed on that specific channel(s).

Taking pressure from the lower back

If there is *pain* with the patient lying on their front, place a *pillow* underneath the patient's waist to take *pressure* away from the *spine*.

Prone position

- With the patient lying face down in a relaxed prone position, begin by relaxing the tissues of the back and legs by using **Mo Fa**, followed by **Gun Fa** and **Rou Fa**.

- Use **Gun Fa** on the glutes, followed by **An Fa/Ya Fa** with the elbow to stimulate GB-30 (Huan Tiao).

- Use **Gun Fa** down the legs, followed by **Rou Fa** with the forearm to relax the tissues. If there is a lot of tension in the hamstrings, bend the knee to shorten the tissues and disengage the muscles. Use **Ji Fa** sporadically to encourage circulation of Qi and Blood.

- Use **Na Fa** on the hamstrings and moving down to the calf, followed by stimulating BL-40 (Wei Zhong) and BL-57 (Cheng Shan) with **An Fa** or **Yi Zhi Chan Tui Fa**.

- Ask the patient to move one leg to the side, in an army crawl position, and use **Mo Fa** followed by **Gun Fa** and **Rou Fa** to relax the Gall Bladder Sinew channel, then return the leg to its normal position. Repeat this on both sides.

- Use **Rou Fa** with the thumb to stimulate K-3 (Tai Xi) and BL-60 (Kun Lun).

- Use **Dou Fa** and **Yao Fa** on both legs at the same time to help release the Sinew channels of the legs and lower back.

Supine position

- Ask the patient to turn over and lie in a relaxed supine position. Use **Mo Fa**, followed by **Gun Fa** and **Rou Fa** on the thigh aspect of the Stomach Sinew channel.

- Use **Yao Fa** on the hips, followed by **Ba Shen Fa** on the hips and lower back.

Prone position

- Ask the patient to again turn over, and move back up to the back and use **Tui Fa** across the Bladder Sinew channel followed by **An Fa** to stimulate the Hua Tuo Jia Ji points of the vertebra from the mid back to the sacrum.

- Use **Gun Fa** on the mid back and lumbar aspect of the Bladder Sinew channel.

- If there is restriction of the lumbar vertebra, use **Gun Fa** and **Tui Fa** to further relax the lumbar area, followed by **Ban Fa** on the lower back. If there is subluxation of the sacro-iliac joint, use **Gun Fa** and **Rou Fa** on the sacrum, followed by **Ban Fa** on the sacrum and **Yao Fa** on the lower back.

- Finish with **Tui Fa** down the legs to dredge the channels, and **Pai Fa** in the lumbar region and hamstrings to disperse Qi and Blood.

Treatment of the upper limbs

Before any specific treatment of the upper limbs is carried out, it is important that work has been done on the neck and shoulders. This is primarily to allow for a better flow of

Qi and Blood into the limbs in order to facilitate healing. As mentioned previously, this is because it is necessary for the Qi Men (gateways) to be fully open, and the neck and the shoulders are the main gateways to the upper limbs. What's more, all three of the Yang arm Sinew channels converge at DU-14 (Da Zhui), so work on this region is vital to release the tissues of the upper limbs. The following sequence is a basic example of how to work on the neck and shoulders before any upper limb treatment is performed.

Seated position

- With the patient in a relaxed seated position, begin with **Mo Fa** to relax the upper back and shoulders on both sides, followed by alternating between **Gun Fa** and **Rou Fa**.

- Use **Fen Tui Fa** across the upper back across the Bladder Sinew channel, followed by **Na Fa** on the trapezius muscles.

- With one hand on the patient's forehead to take pressure and tension from the neck muscles, use **Na Fa** on the nape of the neck from the occiput down to the base of the neck. Use **Gun Fa** from the shoulders into the neck for 2–3 minutes each side.

- Stimulate GB-20 (Feng Chi) and GB-21 (Jian Jing) with **An Fa**.

- Support the arm with one hand in a horizontal position, and use **Gun Fa** into the shoulder joint, followed by gentle **Ba Shen Fa** to open up the shoulder.

- Stimulate SI-9 (Jian Zhen) at the back of the shoulder with **An Fa**.

- If necessary, perform **Ban Fa** on the lower neck and upper back, with a focus on mobilising C7 and T1.

Prone position

- Ask the patient to lie face down in a prone position, and use **Gun Fa** and **Rou Fa** to further relax the muscles of the shoulders and upper back.

- Use **Tui Fa** across the neck aspect of the Bladder Sinew channel, followed by gentle **Na Fa**.

- Finish with **Ji Fa** and **Pai Fa** on the upper back and shoulder to stimulate the flow of Qi and Blood.

General shoulder pain

Shoulder injuries are common, and can be tricky to treat due to the complex nature of the shoulder joint, and the amount of channels that engage the shoulder. For any shoulder injury, it is important to work on the scapula region of the Small Intestine Sinew channel no matter what – being the arm aspect of the Tai Yang Sinew channels, almost all movement of the shoulder originates with movement of the scapular. This is why fully mobilising the scapular by working on the Small Intestine Sinew channel is absolutely vital to hold the shoulder correctly in place, and to allow fully functional movement. In addition to this, identification of the affected Sinew channel(s) is important to understand what is causing dysfunction or discomfort of the shoulder, and working along the full channel is usually necessary.

The shoulder

The *shoulder* is a very *complex* joint that is essentially floating, being only supported by a number of *Sinew channels* and *tissue structures* rather than any major bone structure. This is due to the fact that the 'ball' of the humerus is actually much bigger than the 'socket' of the shoulder blade. This makes the shoulder one of the most *mobile joints* in the body, although unfortunately, one of the most troublesome. Often, treatment of the shoulder will involve *multiple Sinew channels*.

For the treatment of general shoulder pain, incorporate the following procedure into the basic sequence on the neck and shoulder discussed previously.

Seated position

- Whilst supporting the patient's arm with one hand and making slight movements using **Yao Fa**, use **Gun Fa** along the deltoid and scapular aspect of the Small Intestine Sinew channel.

- Whilst still supporting the patient's arm, use **Tui Fa** across the upper arm and shoulder joint (both anteriorly and posteriorly) for 3–4 minutes, followed by **Na Fa**.

- Use **Cuo Fa** on the shoulder joint and down the arm, followed by **Dou Fa**.

- Stimulate the Small Intestine Jing Well point, in addition to other Jing Well points of the affected channel(s) using **An Fa**. Follow this with using **An Fa** or **Yi Zhi Chan Tui Fa** on GB-21 (Jian Jing).

- Use **Yao Fa** to rotate and rock the shoulder joint, followed by **Ba Shen Fa** to open up the joint and increase the circulation of Qi and Blood through the joint.

- Finish off with **Pai Fa** and **Ji Fa** on the upper back.

Supine position

- Ask the patient to lie face up in a relaxed supine position. Hold and support the arm of the affected side with one hand, whilst using the other hand to perform **Rou Fa** and **Gun Fa** into the front of shoulder joint, focusing on the Large Intestine and Lung Sinew channels.

- After 1–2 minutes, begin to rock and rotate the arm using **Yao Fa** with the supporting hand in a comfortable arc (within the patient's range of movement), whilst still using **Rou Fa** and **Gun Fa**.

- Use **Gun Fa** along the upper arm and chest aspects of the Lung Sinew channel to help open up the shoulder joint.

Prone position

- Ask the patient to lie face down in a relaxed prone position, and use **Gun Fa**, **Rou Fa** and **Tui Fa** on the back and neck aspects of the Small Intestine and Bladder Sinew channels.

- Use **Yao Fa** to move and mobilise the scapular, followed by **An Fa** or **Yi Zhi Chan Tui Fa** on SI-11 (Tian Zong) and each of the Hua Tuo Jia Ji points of the thoracic vertebrae.

- Finish off using **Pai Fa** and **Ji Fa**.

General elbow pain

Most elbow issues present as what Western medical science would call medial epicondylitis (known as golfer's elbow), or lateral epicondylitis (known as tennis elbow). These affect the Yin Sinew channels and Yang Sinew channels respectively. Although treatment of each one is similar, there should be a focus on either the Yin channels or Yang channels depending on which are being affected. Otherwise, treatment principles will be the same.

Once the basic sequence for the upper limbs has been done, use the following procedure for the treatment of general elbow pain.

Seated position

- Begin with **Cuo Fa** and **Na Fa** on the major muscles of the upper arm to help open the channels leading into the elbow.

- Use **Tui Fa** across the channels from the elbow to the wrist, followed by pushing with **Tui Fa** from the wrist back up towards the elbow. Repeat this nine times.

- Use **Rou Fa** to stimulate key points around the elbow, focusing on LI-10 (Shou San Li), LI-11 (Qu Chi) and SJ-10 (Tian Jing) for the Yang channels, or H-3 (Shou Hai) and P-3 (Qu Ze) for the Yin channels.

- Use **Na Fa** on the main muscle bellies of the forearm.

- Once the forearm is relaxed, use **Tan Bo Fa** along the affected Sinew channels followed by gentle **Rou Fa** with the thumb along each channel from the elbow to the wrist to help reduce any stagnation.

- Use **Yao Fa** at both the shoulder and elbow to mobilise the joints.

- Use **Ba Shen Fa** on the wrist and fingers, and **Nian Fa** and **An Fa** to stimulate the Jing Well points of the channels associated with the elbow pain.

General wrist pain

Once the basic sequence on upper limbs has been done, perform the above sequence for the elbow to open up the joint and relax the forearm, then use the following procedure for the treatment of general wrist pain. The same procedure may be used for carpal tunnel syndrome.

Seated position

- Use **Rou Fa** with the thumb to stimulate key points around the wrist, such as SJ-4 (Yang Chi), P-7 (Da Ling), LI-5 (Yang Xi) and SI-5 (Yang Gu).

- Use **Fen Tui Fa** across the palm root of the hand, followed by **Gui Tui Fa** on the major and minor thenar eminence.

- Use **Yao Fa** and gentle **Ba Shen Fa** on the wrist joint, followed by each of the fingers joints. Use **Nian Fa** on each finger and the first and fifth metacarpals up to the wrist joint.

- Use **Tan Bo Fa** across the major tendons travelling through the wrist joint, followed by **Rou Fa** from the wrist towards the elbow.

- Strongly stimulate LI-10 (Shou San Li) and H-3 (Shou Hai) with **An Fa** or **Rou Fa** with the thumb, followed by gentle **Dou Fa**. (This should be gentle so that it does not put too much force through the wrist joint.)

Treatment of the lower limbs

Before any specific treatment of the lower limbs is carried out, it is important that work has been done on the lower back and hips in order to allow for better flow of Qi and Blood into the lower limbs. As mentioned previously, this is because it is important to ensure that the Qi Men (gateways) are fully open for healing to properly take place. The lower back and hips are the main gateways to the lower limbs, with the knees also acting as gateways to the ankles. A basic procedure to release the lower back and hips may be as follows.

Prone position

- With the patient lying on their front in a relaxed prone position, begin with **Mo Fa** and **Rou Fa** on the mid and lower back, followed by **Gun Fa** to release the Bladder Sinew channel.

- Use **Tui Fa** across the Bladder Sinew channel at the lower back, followed again by **Gun Fa** moving towards the glutes and hamstrings.

- Use **Rou Fa** with the forearm on the glutes and hamstrings to relax the tissues, followed by **Ya Fa** with the forearm/elbow on GB-30 (Huan Tiao) for 4–5 seconds. If the tissues are particularly tight, bend the patient's knee and hold their lower leg at a slight angle to help release tension in the upper leg and glutes.

- Use **Rou Fa**, **Gun Fa** and **Ji Fa** to relax and open the Sinew channels on the hamstrings.

- Ask the patient to bend their knee and bring their leg to the side (in an army crawl-type position) to get better access to the Gall Bladder Sinew channels, and use **Gun Fa** and **Rou Fa** along the side of the leg, focusing at the hip by the glutes and into the sacrum.

- Ask the patient to return to a comfortable prone position with one leg bent at a 90-degree angle. Place one hand in a fist position in the region of GB-30 (Huan Tiao) and take hold of the patient's ankle with the other hand. Strongly perform **Ya Fa** with the fist into GB-30 (Huan Tiao) at the same time as pulling the ankle towards you. Repeat this three times.

- Perform **Ba Shen Fa** on the lower back and hips to open up the Qi Men, followed by **Yao Fa** on the hips and lower back. This can be performed with the patient lying in either a supine or prone position, although it is often easier in a supine position.

- Finish off by using **Ji Fa** and **Pai Fa** down the whole Bladder Sinew channel, starting at the mid back followed by dredging the channel with **Tui Fa** three times.

General knee pain

As with any joint, it is first necessary to relax and open up the Sinew channels that flow through the region. This is particularly important with regards to the knee in order to open up the spaces within the knee joint to allow the Qi and Blood to flow freely in and out of the area. The knees suffer a lot from compaction due to the constant forces being transferred through the joint. Although the knees should *transfer* force rather than *bear* force, due to poor posture and body movements, the knees often absorb a lot of compression and force into the joint.

When treating the knee, time should first be spent working on *all* Sinew channels that run through the knee. This would be the Bladder, Gall Bladder, Stomach, Spleen, Kidney and Liver Sinew channels. Once the basic sequence to open up the lower limbs has been done, use the following procedure for the treatment of general knee pain.

Supine position

- With the patient lying in a relaxed supine position, begin with **Mo Fa** and **Gun Fa** on the thigh for 4–5 minutes.

- Use **Tui Fa** across the Stomach Sinew channel followed by the Spleen Sinew channel just above the knee, in the region of SP-10 (Xue Hai) and ST-34 (Liang Qiu), followed by a combined technique of **Na Fa** and **Dou Fa**.

- Ask the patient to bend their knee and rotate their leg outwards, creating a 'figure of four' shape with their legs – this helps to expose the Yin Sinew channels of the upper leg. Use **Gun Fa** and **Rou Fa** to relax the channels.

- Use **Ba Shen Fa** on the knee two to three times, increasing pressure each time, followed by strong **An Fa** into the eyes of the knee for 4–5 seconds.

- With the knee up, bent at 90 degrees, use **Cuo Fa** on the lower leg focusing on releasing and relaxing the calf muscle. Strongly stimulate ST-36 (Zu San Li) and GB-34 (Yang Ling Quan) with **An Fa** or **Rou Fa**.

- Position the knee into a straight position again and use **Tui Fa** across the patella tendon.

Prone position

- Ask the patient to turn over and lie face down in a relaxed prone position. Begin with using **Gun Fa** on the thigh aspect of the Bladder Sinew channel, followed by using **Rou Fa** with the forearm for extra pressure – if there is a lot of tension in the muscles, bend the leg slightly to shorten and slacken the tissues so that you can get deeper into the channels.

- To avoid stagnation from strong techniques, use **Ji Fa** intermittently between techniques to encourage the circulation of Qi and Blood.

- Use **Tui Fa** to push up the calf aspect of the Bladder Sinew channel, followed by **Tui Fa** across the Bladder Sinew channel.

- Use **Tan Bo Fa** on the tendons behind the knee and at GB-34 (Yang Ling Quan), followed by **Mo Fa** to help with any potential stagnation caused by **Tan Bo Fa**.

- Use **Na Fa** on the calf and upper thigh, followed by stimulating any Ashi points on the hamstrings or calf with **An Fa** and BL-40 (Wei Zhong) with **Yi Zhi Chan Tui Fa**.

- With the knee bent and the lower leg in a vertical position, use **Yao Fa** to rock the knee followed by **Ba Shen Fa** on the knee by placing one arm behind the knee and pushing the patient's heel towards their glutes.

- Use **Yao Fa** to rotate the ankle and ensure unrestricted mobility. If there is any restriction in the ankle, follow parts of the ankle routine below.

- Use **Pai Fa** and **Ji Fa** along the whole leg, followed by **Tui Fa** down the whole leg to dredge the channels.

General ankle pain (including plantar fasciitis)

Like the knee, the ankle takes a lot of pressure from day to day, and often suffers from compression and tension around the joint. For this reason, **Ba Shen Fa** and **Yao Fa** are key techniques to help with non-specific ankle pain. However, before performing **Ba Shen Fa**, it is important to establish that there is no instability of the ankle (such as giving way), as it may cause more problems if performed on an unstable joint.

It is also important when treating the ankle that the knee is functional, and that the channels of the whole leg are open before focusing on the foot. This allows for a better circulation of Qi and Blood through the leg, and both in and out of the foot. In fact, when treating foot and ankle injuries, more time is often spent on the leg with only the final parts of treatment being focused directly on the foot. It would be wise to explain this to your patient as they may feel that the treatment has been focused on the incorrect area.

Once the basic sequence to open the lower back has been done, use the following procedure for the treatment of general ankle pain.

Prone position

- With the patient lying face down in a prone position, use **Gun Fa** and **Rou Fa** on the upper leg aspect of the Bladder Sinew channel, followed by **An Fa** or **Ya Fa** on BL-36 (Cheng Fu) and BL-37 (Yin Men) to open up the leg above the knee.

- Gently use **Tan Bo Fa** on the tendons behind the knee, followed by **Na Fa** and **Tui Fa** down the whole leg. Finish with **Tan Bo Fa** and **Na Fa** on the Achilles tendon.

Supine position

- Ask the patient to turn over to lie face up in a supine position. Use **Tui Fa** up the lower leg aspects of the Stomach, Gall Bladder, Spleen and Liver Sinew channels, followed by **Cuo Fa** down the lower leg nine times. Strongly stimulate ST-36 (Zu San Li) with **An Fa** to increase circulation of Qi and Blood to the foot.

- Stimulate GB-40 (Qiu Xu), SP-5 (Shang Qiu) and ST-41 (Jie Xi) with **An Fa** or **Rou Fa** with the thumb. Stimulate specific Jing Well points according to the channel(s) affected with a combination of **Nian Fa** and **An Fa**.

- Use **Tan Bo Fa** across the tendons below K-6 (Zhao Hai) and BL-62 (Shen Mai), and finish with **Ba Shen Fa** (unless the ankle is unstable) and **Yao Fa** to help mobilise the ankle.

- If the patient is suffering from plantar fasciitis, once the above sequence has been done, use **Gui Tui Fa** on the sole of the foot, followed by **Gun Fa** for 4–5 minutes. Finish with **Fen Tui Fa** and **Ji Fa** on the sole of the foot.

Index